TELe-Health

Series editors
Fabio Capello
Cumberland Infirmary
North Cumbria University Hospitals
Carlisle, United Kingdom

Giovanni Rinaldi
Ospedali Riuniti Marche Nord
Pesaro, Italy

Giovanna Gatti
European Institute of Oncology (IEO)
Milan, Italy

Recent advances in technology and medicine are rapidly changing the face of health care. A revolution is occurring in diagnosis and treatment thanks to the implementation of instrumentation and techniques deriving from engineering and research. In addition, a cultural conversion is taking place in which geographical and social boundaries are about to be overcome, resulting in enhanced availability and quality of care. Telemedicine has been considered a possible means of improving health care worldwide that is likely to change the way in which doctors deal with patients and diseases. While various restraints continue to limit the application of telemedicine in different settings and different areas of health, the innovations emerging from eHealth and telecare could stimulate a great leap forward for medicine, provided that some basic rules are taken into consideration and followed.In this series, diverse aspects of tele-health – preventive, promotive, and curative – will be covered by leading experts in the field with the aim of realizing the full potential of the new and exciting technological solutions at our disposal.

More information about this series at http://www.springer.com/series/11892

Multidisciplinary Teleconsultation in Developing Countries

Michelangelo Bartolo · Fabio Ferrari

Editors

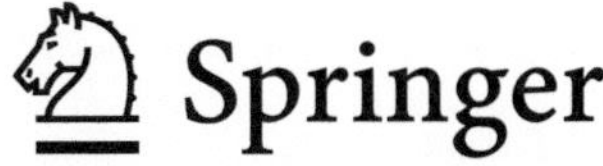 Springer

Editors
Michelangelo Bartolo
Telemedicine Unit
San Giovanni Hospital
Rome, Italy

Fabio Ferrari
University of Rome 'La Sapienza'
Rome, Italy

ISSN 2198-6037   ISSN 2198-6045   (electronic)
TELe-Health
ISBN 978-3-319-72762-2   ISBN 978-3-319-72763-9   (eBook)
https://doi.org/10.1007/978-3-319-72763-9

Library of Congress Control Number: 2018933390

This Springer imprint is published by the registered company Springer International Publishing AG part of Springer Nature.
The registered company address is: Gewerbestrasse 11, 6330 Cham, Switzerland

Foreword

Nowadays, globalisation is perceived as something negative, an inevitable evil that creates inequality, and something that nobody seems to be able to avoid. Consequently, anything that brings people together and lets them communicate with each other is seen as suspicious. Threats such as an increase in the migration flows and the spread of terrorism, which appear to be encouraged by globalisation itself, only increase people's fear.

The reality is actually more complex than that. History, for example, is full of periods of migration, like those involving Italy, between 1800 and 1900. Likewise, there have been other times of terror, even in recent European history.

Nonetheless, there is another aspect of globalisation, which is related to the development of technology, infrastructures, connections and greater accessibility. This is the case of the improvement of the global health service which has come about through the opportunities offered by new forms of advanced communication. In this way, high-income and technologically developed countries could offer support to those left behind, making life in poor-resource settings easier at a relatively low cost. Helping people in their own countries would give one reason less for them to leave their home.

This book in fact deals with the creation of technological networks to be used for training and health. In technical terms, this is called "telemedicine"; it offers "best practices" through connections between places that are very far away from each other—a sort of globalisation of medicine. This subject is fully discussed in the following pages: it is a way to create a new form of international cooperation through technology, which will bring a future and development not only to the countries that benefit from it directly but to both sides of the network.

Until 2011, there had been a decrease in the Italian commitment to International Cooperation in Africa. In the 1990s and in the 2000s, donations were significantly lower compared to the previous decades; sub-Saharan Africa was particularly affected by that. During these years, support to Africa was granted mainly by non-government organizations that received money from the Catholic Church and other religious movements, or from NGOs and government organizations. However, fund-raising for health projects and developing programs became increasingly difficult. In 2012 the trend was reversed and now Italy is again one of the main EU, G7 and OECD donors.

We also changed our approach: in August 2014, a new cooperation law was approved[1] (n. 125), which we had been looking forward to for 20 years. As a result there was the creation of the Development Agency and the possibility for the Deposits and Loans Fund to become an Italian development bank. There was also an expansion in terms of the types of people involved, with the diasporas, the private sector, the non-profit organisations and the non-profit sector in general. This immediately caused an all-round increase in the number of people involved and in the number of projects, and it also heightened the interest of the European Commission. The missions to Africa and the African delegations passing through Rome became far more numerous.

It is not just a matter of renewed Italian interest aiming to increase humanitarian works and projects in some countries that lack infrastructures. Africa has become a strategic priority, as former Italian Prime Minister Matteo Renzi stated during his visit to Mozambique: "an opportunity and not only a continent receiving development assistance".[2] This new strategic presence is the result of having understood that Africa is of strategic value for Italy, for Europe and for the future global geostrategic balance.

Africa has changed too. The continent has grown and there are new opportunities for Italy and for Europe. The presence of activism of China, Turkey, and other Asian countries, which to date is well consolidated, expresses this new global interest in the continent. Africa is a young continent today. Forty-three per cent of the population of sub-Sahara is under 14 years old[3]—a generation born with digital technology—and despite the digital divide, they are perfectly technology savvy. Practically everyone owns a smartphone today, and this can become a vehicle for development and closeness.

During the years, I have been responsible for Italian international cooperation and have visited several excellent health facilities in Africa, set up by many of our NGOs. Last November I went to the Global Health Telemedicine multi-specialist teleconsultation centre in Bangui, Central Africa. With this system, Central African doctors can request and receive any consultation from specialists in the West who are in the network, in real time. Clinical records, admission charts, or consultation notes, together with imaging, and reports from instrumental and laboratory tests are easily accessible and sharable. This allows real-time or delayed consultations offering support for diagnosis and treatment. With this technology, even very poor Central Africa can come out of isolation and benefit from the best treatments. One of the problems with the global medical sector is in fact its separation, which technology

---

[1] http://www.gazzettaufficiale.it/eli/id/2014/08/28/14G00130/sg

[2] http://www.huffingtonpost.it/2016/05/18/conferenza-italia-africa_n_10024618.html

[3] https://www.internazionale.it/opinione/nicolo-cavalli/2015/08/20/africa-economia-sviluppo

can overcome, and the same technology can be used to provide data that is useful for medicine in rich countries.

Everything described in these pages is scientifically based; it is not just a series of success stories in health cooperation but it represents a model that can be replicated in other geographical contexts and, why not, even in our countries. I visited many DREAM centres (in Mozambique, Malawi, Tanzania, etc.) and people with HIV who started living again. I also met motivated, well-trained African health staff, with career prospects, precisely because they can operate within a network and use the best instruments and devices. These are Italian projects that express not only a new health model that consists of the highest quality treatment and diagnostics but also warmth, support, development and training.

A while ago, the Health Minister of Guinea, a doctor, told me unhappily that all the students who graduated from African universities ended up working in European hospitals. I realised that it was not just for the salary: if a recently graduated African student expects to be isolated from the continuous cycle of research, which is particularly true in medicine, he will go where the information is. So how can you keep healthcare in Africa at a level of excellence and also hold on to its doctors? Technology can solve this problem by creating a global network. The network of exchanges and contacts that are created through the thorough application of tele-medicine represents a form of long-distance training, as well as an exchange of data and research. This provides dignity and increases the scientific knowledge and awareness on both sides: health models that are integrated and can spread and grow.

It is not true that poor healthcare is enough for Africa because Africa is poor: the experiences described in this book show that there is only one kind of healthcare and only one kind of health, that is, for everyone.

Rome, Italy

Mario Giro
Deputy Foreign Minister
Responsible for
International Cooperation

Foreword

The richest and most developed countries in the world have a series of services for their many daily healthcare needs that are extremely evolved, although they do have their limits and problems. They reach almost all the population, and in general they also create an element of social stability. We are so used to them that we do not even ask ourselves how they are set up, how much they cost and what it takes to keep them going. We just use them; that's all. In more advanced healthcare systems, like in Italy, we are able to make treatments and assistance, involving considerably complex technological and organisational aspects, easily accessible. One example is the fact that in some Italian regions, it is even possible to have a blood sample taken at home; it is taken immediately and safely to a laboratory that operates within the regional health service. The laboratory performs the blood test and records the information in the region's computer systems, the administrative work is carried out and the laboratory is then paid through an electronic bank transfer. People who use this service can receive their results in just a few hours and forward them to their doctor in real time in the Internet. This all appears to be quite natural to them. Actually this service works, thanks to this complex system that absorbs considerable economic resources and requires that the infrastructures involved be working perfectly, like the electric power distribution and the Internet connection networks.

Unfortunately, systems like this are not yet practical in developing countries, like those of sub-Saharan Africa. There are many reasons for this, but it is mainly because of the lack of resources that has obstructed the evolution of the infrastructures and the distribution networks (of drugs, biomedical products, instruments, etc.). It is therefore difficult for healthcare organisations to be set up throughout the whole country, and progress in the use of digital technologies is very limited. Then the healthcare facilities, most of which are private, do not collaborate with each other to create an organised system, so they are unable to carry out effective prevention and provide continuing assistance.

In order to look at this in realistic terms, one can consider the idea of moving the whole laboratory of our example above to one of these countries. If it were handed over to the people who live there, they would not be able to make the services work on their own. In fact they would not be able to provide the necessary infrastructures and supplies, which in developed countries are considered routine and in fact do involve routine activities. They would not have, for example, efficient electric power supply networks to avoid the malfunctioning of any of the sophisticated electronic laboratory systems. Neither would they have enough qualified technicians to take care of the maintenance of the equipment and repairing breakdowns. Moreover, the Internet connections would be unstable and not even be available in every part of the country.

In the poorest countries, these issues concern all the healthcare activities, both the most basic ones and even more so the highly technological activities, such as telemedicine. So it looks as though it would be very difficult to set up telemedicine services and impossible to keep them running efficiently, in the very places that would benefit from them most.

The benefit of the collaboration between the DREAM project of the Community of Sant'Egidio and the Global Health Telemedicine (GHT) non-profit organisation is that it proposed an effective solution to the above-mentioned problems, which can be maintained over time, and this solution has already been successfully set up in several countries in Africa. In fact, by using the features of telemedicine and the brilliant innovations in terms of the IT processes, the DREAM and GHT network, in collaboration with the local authorities, is able to overcome these apparently unre-solvable issues, and it also covers the costs of setting up and running all the necessary IT systems. With extensive telemonitoring and clinical teleconsultation services, this network makes it possible for the African healthcare staff to use biomedical devices and receive specialist medical consulting free of charge.

What has made it possible to achieve this extremely valuable result is basically the fact that the whole telemedicine system was designed and set up with the very highest clinical standards. This is why the Italian Society of Digital Health and Telemedicine is actively promoting the DREAM and GHT platform, which has already been supported by authoritative Italian experts, and is looking forward to and encouraging a more and more extensive use of this solution.

Another interesting aspect of this solution is that the teleconsultation activities performed by the GHT network have made it possible to increase the collaboration between Italian experts and local health staff.

The local health staff obviously had to be trained to be able to use the digital instruments and become familiar with the innovations in the processes used. On the other hand, the Italian GHT Teleconsultation specialists sometimes found them-selves dealing with severe clinical situations, without being able to resort to sophis-ticated diagnostic instruments. They had to rely on simple rural healthcare centres, maybe run by just one nurse, for the advice they gave regarding diagnosis and treatment. This was a new situation that the specialists, although experts in their field, had to quickly learn to cope with, from both a technical and a human point of view, in order to "rethink" their operative clinical responses.

It was a question of directing the therapeutic solutions towards the good practices they are used to and of finding solutions that could be applied in the local context.

This involved a process of adapting to "feasible" clinical work in situations with extremely limited resources, which made the results achieved even more exciting.

The telemedicine system set up by GHT is efficient from an economic and organisational point of view and effective from a clinical point of view. It is versatile in that it can be used in different situations and geographic areas, and it contributes to the progress of developing countries by providing training for local healthcare staff.

The GHT programme therefore guarantees a new form of healthcare cooperation with a high impact and low cost, and it eliminates the distance between specialists and patients.

We hope that the Italian National Health System will also be able to benefit from this experience. Now that the experimental phase is finally over, this seems to be the right time to develop operational support for healthcare activities in various contexts, making them consistent and accessible. The experiences described in this book represent the concrete proof that when the procedures are streamlined, this is perfectly feasible.

We greatly appreciate this book and its operational context, and we believe that projects like this can demonstrate how essential telemedicine is in ensuring high-quality healthcare activities for everyone. What has been done in a precarious organisational context with limited infrastructures can certainly be planned and set up in well-organised places with adequate infrastructures, like in Italy with our National Health System.

So this is a great opportunity for our readers to find out about a revolutionary vision.

Digital SIT – Italian Society for Digital Health   Gianfranco Gensini
and Telemedicine
Rome, Italy

National Centre for Telemedicine and
New Healthcare Technologies
Italian National Health Institute
Rome, Italy

Digital SIT – Italian Society for Digital Health   Francesco Gabbrielli
and Telemedicine
Rome, Italy

National Centre for Telemedicine and
New Healthcare Technologies
Italian National Health Institute
Rome, Italy

Acknowledgments

San Giovanni Hospital, Rome, Italy
University of Tor Vergata, Rome, Italy
Nico I Frutti del Chicco—Onlus, Rome, Italy
Luconlus—non-profit humanitarian association, Rome, Italy
ScudoMed, non-profit association, Rome, Italy
Apurimac—non-profit association, Rome, Italy
Amici del Centrafrica—Onlus, Limido Comasco, Como,Italy
Rotary Club Rome, Italy
Rotary International, Italy
Foundation I.R.C.S.S. (Scientific Institutes of Hospitalization an care) Neurological
    Institute "Carlo Besta", Milan, Italy
Fondation "Arpa", Pisa, Italy
S. Camillo Forlanini Hospital, Rome, Italy
Rome Airports—ADR, Italy
University Hospital "A. Gemelli", Rome, Italy
Pediatric Hospital "Bambino Gesù", Rome, Italy
Ttre Information Communication Technology, Rome, Italy
Caroline Swinton—mother tongue translator, Rome, Italy

Luigi Badaloni
Claudio Benedetti
Gaetano Biafora
Antonietta Capozzi
Gabriele Cirilli
Luisa Cordova
Antonio D'Alessandro
Francesco De Giorgi
Agostino De Girolamo
Andrea De Santis
Maria Di Vietro
Tommaso Gargallo
Elisabetta Gennaro
Gianpiero Guerrieri

Rino Maisto
Simone Mastrostefano
Grigorij Mele
Andrea Mezzanzanica
Mauro Mocci
Paolo Mori
Chiara Pierri
Chiara Razzi Di Nunzio
Giuseppe Repole
Matteo Rizzolli
Patrizia Ruscio
Giuseppe Quintavalle
Antonio Segatori
Giovanni Tortorolo
Vincenzo Viggiani
Paola Zabini

We thank all the doctors who collaborate as voluntary and referring doctors.
We thank the donors who support the telemedicine services.

In memory
Giorgio Scaffidi
Enrico Fraschetti

Introduction

We live in a world in which divisions, particularism and ethnicism lead to an increase in the number of walls and barriers. In 1989, with the fall of the Berlin wall, it looked as though the world was at the beginning of a new era in which the divisions and barriers were going to disappear. Today, 25 years later, there are 70 walls dividing countries, which is 47 more than before, and more walls are likely to be built in the future.

These are real, concrete barriers, but maybe even more than that, they are cultural barriers that increase the distance between a rich world and many countries that live in obviously difficult conditions.

Considering this situation, the cross-border telemedicine services[4] discussed in this book do not only represent an undeniably useful healthcare service; they can also be a bridge that crosses those sometimes insurmountable walls and creates proximity and training.

One aspect of healthcare cooperation that is sometimes not taken into account is that it brings together populations that are physically and culturally far apart.

Teleconsultation and telemonitoring thousands of patients who, because of their geographic location, would otherwise never be able to receive a medical opinion from the best doctors and hospitals not only has positive repercussions on their health but also on their families. Telemedicine also provides benefits for the local healthcare staff who, even though they work in unstable conditions, with just a click are able to reach specialists who are prepared to offer a second opinion. This service goes far beyond the albeit high value of a single teleconsultation; it represents a kind of valid continuous long-distance training.

DREAM, of the Community of Sant'Egidio, and Global Health Telemedicine have always aimed to avoid a minimalist approach and to offer excellence not only in their training but also in terms of electromedical devices and laboratory equipment.

---

[4]Italian Ministry of Health. National telemedicine guidelines. 2014—Sect. 8.4.

The DREAM programme was the first cooperation project to take the antiretroviral therapy to Africa, and it introduced the viral load as an essential test for everyone.

In the same way, Global Health Telemedicine has always used latest generation devices, refusing to take equipment that is no longer used in Europe, which used to be donated with the idea that it was "better than nothing".

In conclusion, this book describes not only a successful international project; it does more than that: it is the story of the tenacity of professionals who have invested personally in a dream of development for a village, a town, a country and a continent. These projects are already a point of reference for many people and they can spread to many other countries. In an increasingly globalised world, we have seen that, particularly in the field of healthcare, countries that are far away from each other are connected. One example of this is the mobilisation that came about for the global health Ebola emergency. This was a joint international effort to counter a threat that could easily have spread to other continents. The whole world is closely connected, and thinking that we can isolate ourselves is just an illusion.

This book shows that investing in healthcare cooperation opens possibilities for development, for the future in general, and even for peace.

That is quite something!

Telemedicine Unit, San Giovanni Hospital   Michelangelo Bartolo
Rome, Italy
University of Rome 'La Sapienza'   Fabio Ferrari
Rome, Italy

Contents

Part I

Africa Today

Health in Sub-Saharan Africa: HIV, TB and Malaria Epidemiology

1

Leonardo Palombi and Stefania Moramarco

The health landscape in sub-Saharan Africa continues to be dominated by the three major epidemics: HIV/AIDS, TB and malaria. However, international commitment has produced major changes in epidemic trends and in the burden of the diseases, although much remains to be done. A recent WHO document on *"Accelerating progress on HIV, tuberculosis, malaria, hepatitis and neglected tropical diseases"* stated that *"The massive international response to HIV, tuberculosis (TB) and malaria has markedly reduced global case incidence and mortality rates, and saved over 50 million lives"*. This result was achieved in the past 15 years and represents a successful response to the greatest health challenge of humanity. This result is also a direct consequence of globalization: only concentrated efforts by governments, international agencies, NGOs and universities have allowed an effective response. However, the same document states that "despite this progress, HIV, TB and malaria continue to pose a major public health threat, killing nearly 3 million people every year". In point of fact, it can be added that in recent years the international economic commitment has diminished, as a result of a dangerous slowdown in treatment and prevention plans. However, Sustainable Development Goals (SDGs), and previously Millennium Development Goals (MDGs), do not neglect the impact of these diseases on global health and indeed emphasize with specific health goals their importance in the context of sustainable development: target 3.3 in the SDG calls on the world to end the epidemics of AIDS, TB and malaria by 2030.

L. Palombi (✉) · S. Moramarco
Department of Biomedicine and Prevention, Tor Vergata University, Rome, Italy
e-mail: palombi@uniroma2.it; stefania.moramarco@gmail.com

© Springer International Publishing AG, part of Springer Nature 2018
M. Bartolo, F. Ferrari (eds.), *Multidisciplinary Teleconsultation in Developing Countries*, TELe-Health, https://doi.org/10.1007/978-3-319-72763-9_1

Fig. 1.1 Global trends in HIV, TB and malaria incidence

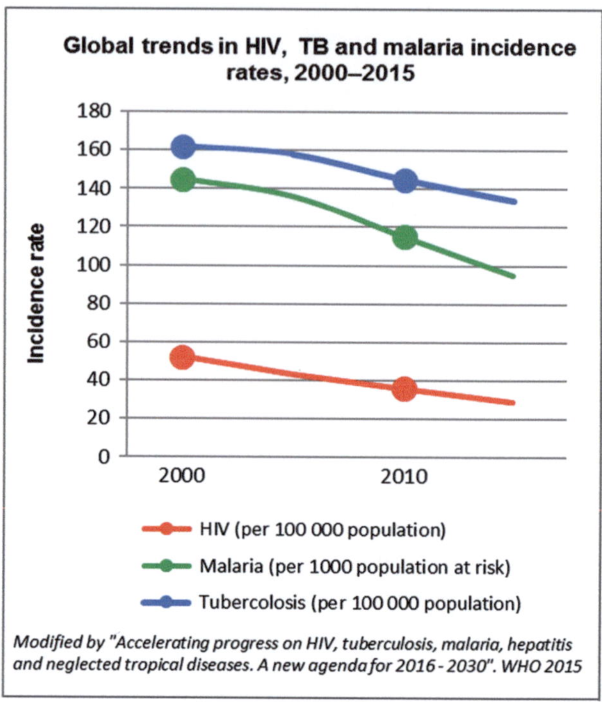

1.1 Global HIV, TB and Malaria Incidence and Mortality Rates

A first analysis deals with the temporal trends of the three major pandemics in the years 2000–2015. Figure 1.1 shows incidence rate data (new cases per year for 100,000 people) of HIV, TB and malaria. Generally, we can see an annual decrease for all the diseases examined, with a more pronounced decline for the HIV/AIDS epidemic. In fact, new cases of HIV dropped from 3.1 million in 2000 to 2.0 million in 2014. The decline in HIV incidence has resulted from fewer children younger than 15 years acquiring HIV, more than 50% less in 2010–2015. This big result has been due to the enormous progress made with prevention of mother-to-child transmission (PMTCT) and paediatric HIV treatment. Since 2000, TB incidence has annually fallen by an average of 1.5%, but the annual decline needs to accelerate to a 4–5% in order to reach the 2020 target of the "End TB Strategy".

Also, HIV-related deaths fell by 24% to 1.2 million in 2014, even among children aged under 15 years: in 2014, 150,000 children were estimated to die of HIV-related causes, 48% fewer than the peak of 290,000 (260,000–320,000) children deaths in 2004. However, the number of people living with HIV rose from an estimated 9.0 million in 1990 to 36.9 million in 2014, due to the rapid scaling up of antiretroviral treatment coverage and the consequent substantial improvement in survival rates.

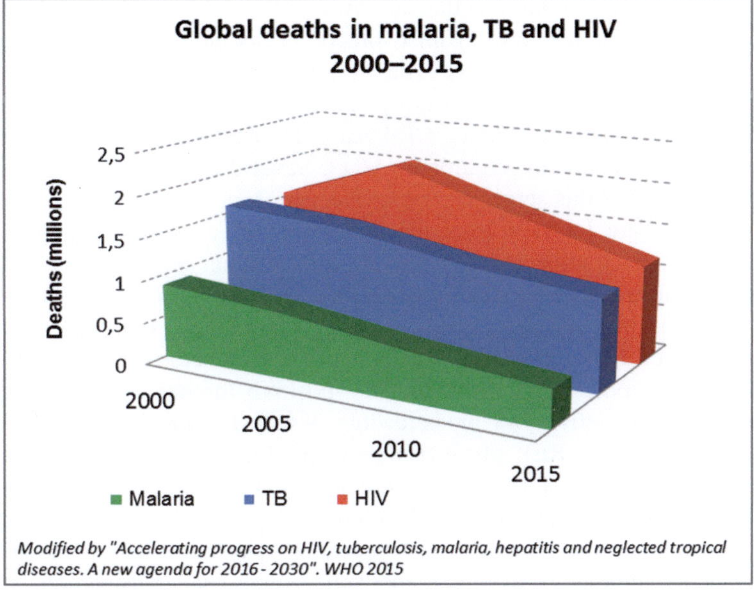

Fig. 1.2 Number of deaths caused by malaria, TB and HIV from 2000 to 2015

Globally, TB incidence fell by an average of 1.5% per year between 2000 and 2014, accounting for a cumulative reduction of 18%. There were an estimated 9.6 million new cases in 2014. The mortality rate fell by 47% worldwide between 1990 and 2015, with most of that improvement occurring during the MDG period.

The malaria mortality rate dropped by 60% between 2000 and 2015, with an estimated 438,000 malaria deaths occurring in 2015. Despite this progress, about 3.2 billion people in 97 countries and territories were still at risk of being infected with malaria in 2015.

The impetus given since 2000 to the fight against HIV has produced complex changes that did not only affect this pandemic, but the whole epidemiological framework. If you look at Fig. 1.2, you can appreciate the changes in mortality rates for HIV, TB and malaria. The decline in HIV and malaria is evident. Numbers of TB-related deaths have slowly decreased in the last years, and in 2015 TB was one of the top 10 causes of death worldwide, ranking above HIV/AIDS as one of the leading causes of death from an infectious disease.

1.2   HIV/AIDS: Epidemiological Perspective

Before proceeding to a more detailed analysis of the epidemiology of the pandemics, it is useful to remember that HIV/AIDS plays a specific role with its immune depressive action.

In fact, the human immunodeficiency virus (HIV) targets the immune system and impairs patient's response against infections (including TB, HPV and many other infectious agents) and cancer. The virus kills specific cells, CD4, deputed to coordinate and activate several immune responses. After 2–15 years from the onset of the infection, the reduction of CD4 leads to the final stage of disease: the acquired immunodeficiency syndrome, AIDS. Several infections and tumours are usually associated at this stage.

There is no cure for HIV infection. However, effective antiretroviral (ARV) drugs can control the virus and help prevent transmission so that people with HIV, and those at substantial risk, can enjoy healthy, long and productive lives.

The infection is transmitted directly, through blood or sexual intercourse. The vast majority of infections in Africa are associated with heterosexual relationships.

The transmission of HIV from an HIV-positive mother to her child during pregnancy, labour, delivery or breastfeeding is called vertical or mother-to-child transmission (MTCT). Risk of vertical transmission ranges from 30% to 45%. Antiretroviral treatment during pregnancy and breastfeeding can effectively prevent the transmission of infection to the child.

These specific characteristics of HIV infection—absence of a cure and need of a lifelong therapy, multiple co-infections and vertical and sexual transmission—required a profound change in African healthcare systems. Indeed, there is a strong need for a highly decentralized healthcare system, dedicated lab diagnostic systems and advanced computerized information system: millions of patients need to be followed not far from the places they live for as long as they live.

It is in this context that we understand the importance of telemedicine, especially if we consider the historical difficulties of access to health services in sub-Saharan Africa.

In 2015 there were globally a total of 36.7 million [34.0 million–39.8 million] people living with HIV. In 2015 there were 2.1 million [1.8 million–2.4 million] new HIV infections worldwide, with almost 1 million people [830.000–1.1 million] living in the world's most affected region, Eastern and Southern Africa. In regions where the gender imbalance is more pronounced, such as sub-Saharan Africa, adolescent girls and young women are at most risk of HIV infection. Figure 1.3 shows the distribution by age and gender in the world and sub-Saharan Africa. You can see the strong impact of the disease on young people and the different sex distribution in Africa with 17% of young women vs 11% in the world. Moreover, women account for 56% of new HIV infections among adults. Strong gender norms against inequalities, right access to education and sexual and reproductive health services and fight against poverty, food insecurity and violence are the crucial weapons to reduce increased HIV risk for young women and adolescent girls.

In the last few years, decline in new HIV infections among adults has slowed alarmingly, with the estimated annual number of new infections among adults, remaining in 2015 nearly static at about 1.9 million [1.7 million–2.2 million], especially when considering new HIV infection in Eastern and Southern Africa. In 2015 a 4% decline has been registered in new adult HIV infections as compared to 2010, about 40,000 fewer new adults HIV infected. At the same time, despite that

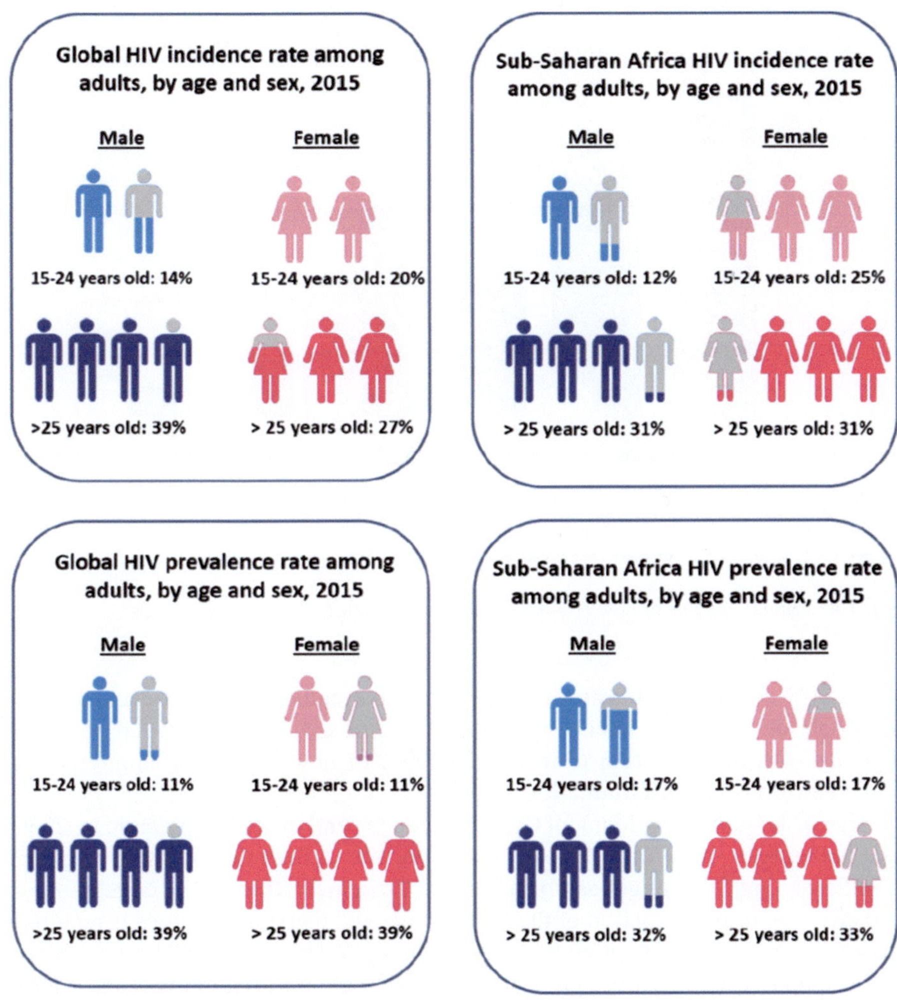

Fig. 1.3 Incidence and prevalence rate at global level and in sub-Saharan African countries

the global number of deaths for HIV-related causes has declined annually, in 2015 still 1.1 million people worldwide [940,000–1.3 million] were dying from HIV-related causes, a number which is by now unacceptable. The global reduction in adult deaths has been greater among women than men (33% vs 15%), reflecting higher treatment coverage among women than men (52% vs 41%).

There is therefore a strong need to rapidly reduce the number of new HIV infections and the number of people dying for HIV-related causes, in order to meet the fast-track target by 2020 (Fig. 1.4). The fast-track targets include the 90-90-90 treatment target (90% of people living with HIV knowing their HIV

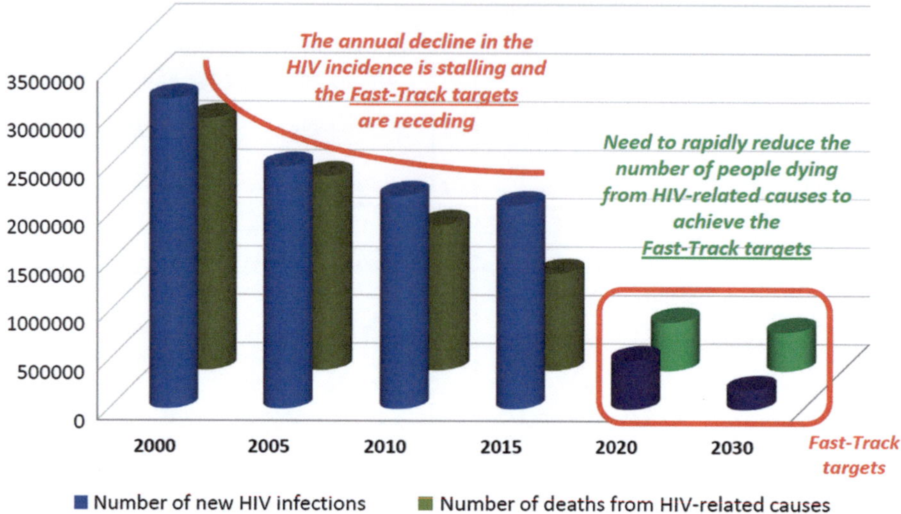

Fig. 1.4 Annual number of new HIV infection and death from HIV-related causes

status, 90% of people who know their HIV-positive status accessing treatment, 90% of people on treatment having viral loads suppressed) to be achieved by 2020, together with the reduction (down to 500,000) of new infections among adults, while ensuring zero discrimination.

The Sustainable Development Goals include the end of AIDS epidemic by 2030, as a bold target. In the last 15 years, many steps have been taken, inspiring global confidence that SDG target can be achieved. To achieve this global target, a rapid and effective implementation of the WHO "treat all" recommendations is required. Countries are rapidly adopting and implementing WHO "treat all" policies along with supportive HIV testing, prevention and strategic information policies. "Treat all" strategies contain key recommendations to treat people living with HIV, including children, adolescents, adults, pregnant and breastfeeding women and people with co-infections.

HIV treatment is essential to save millions more lives, especially since HIV treatment is getting increasingly affordable and effective. For example, compared to HIV transmission rates of 15–45% when mothers and infants are untreated, PMTCT reduces this rate below 5%. By the end of 2014, about 73% of pregnant women worldwide living with HIV had received ARVs as part of PMTCT, up from 53% in 2009 and just 1% in 2000.

The goal of providing HIV treatment to 15 million people by the end of 2015 was achieved. In 2015 the number of people living with HIV on antiretroviral therapy

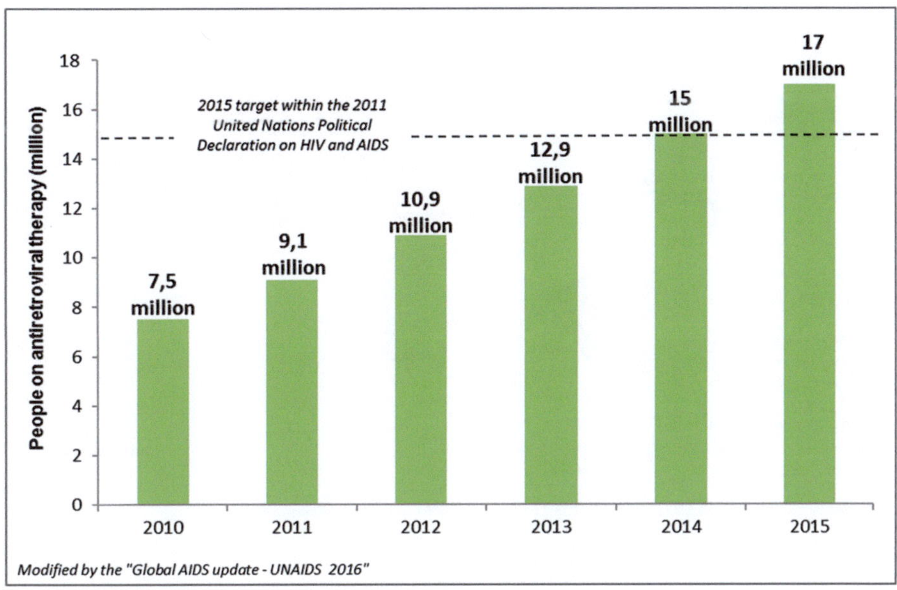

Fig. 1.5 Global number of people living with HIV on antiretroviral therapy, 2010–2015

reached 17.0 million people, about 2 million more than the target set by the United Nations General Assembly of 15 million people by 2015 (Fig. 1.5).

Nevertheless, in 2016 more than 18.2 million people [16.1 million–19 million] were estimated to receive HIV treatment, only 46% of the 36.7 million people living globally with HIV in 2015 were receiving ART, and many started treatment when their HIV infection was well advanced.

Better figures were achieved in the Eastern and Southern Africa, the world's most affected region: coverage of antiretroviral therapy rose from 24% in 2010 to 54% in 2015, with totally about 10.3 million people receiving antiretroviral therapy (more than doubled in the last 5 years). South Africa alone had nearly 3.4 million people on treatment, more than any other country in the world. After South Africa, Kenya has the largest treatment programme in Africa (nearly 900,000 people on treatment) followed by Botswana, Eritrea, Malawi, Mozambique, Rwanda, Swaziland, Uganda, the United Republic of Tanzania, Zambia and Zimbabwe (treatment coverage increased by more than 25% between 2010 and 2015) (Fig. 1.6).

Figure 1.7 combines the number of HIV-related causes and the number of people receiving ART by year. Globally, the increase in treatment has resulted in a 26% decline in AIDS-related deaths, from an estimated 1.5 million [1.3 million–1.7 million] in 2010 to 1.1 million [940,000–1.3 million] in 2015. AIDS-related deaths have also been reduced in the world's most affected region, Eastern and Southern Africa, having decreased by 36% since 2010.

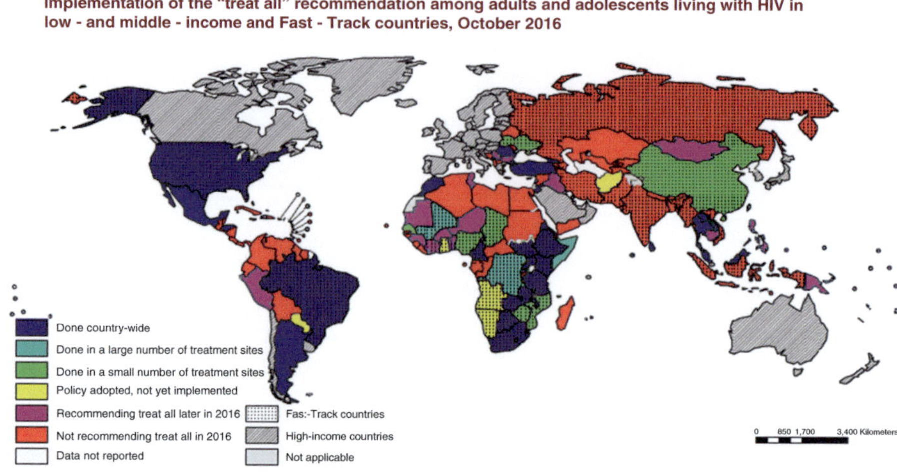

Fig. 1.6 World map of "treat all" implementation, 2016

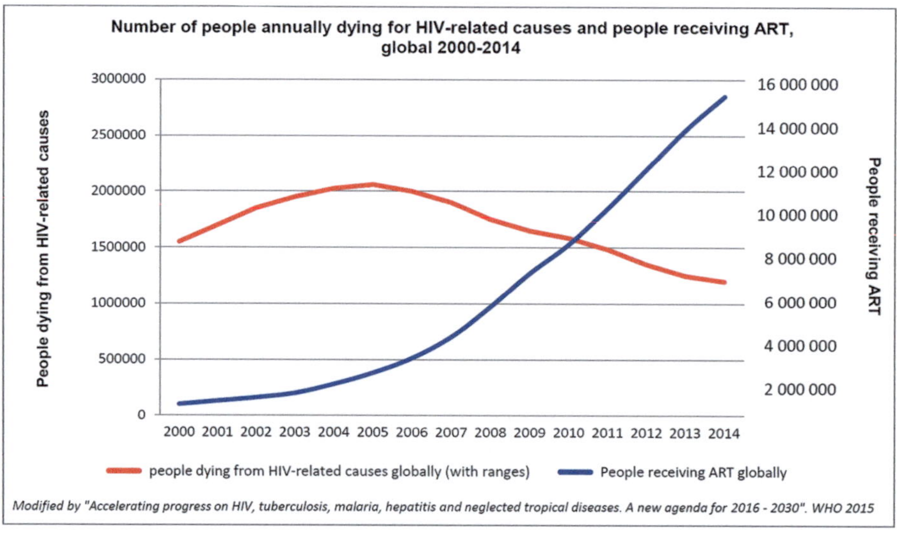

Fig. 1.7 Number of people dying for HIV-related causes and people receiving ART, 2000–2004

1.3 TB: Epidemiological Perspective

Tuberculosis (TB) is caused by bacteria (*Mycobacterium tuberculosis*) that most often affect the lungs and can be spread from person to person through the air.

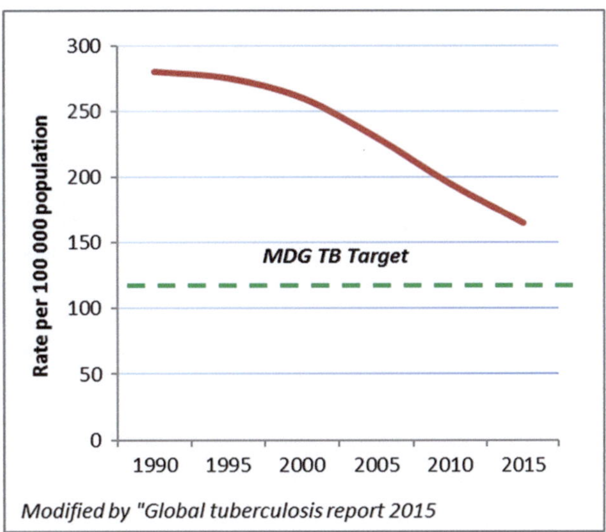

Fig. 1.8 Global TB prevalence rate, 1990–2015

Tuberculosis (TB) is one of the top 10 causes of death worldwide: yet it is a curable and preventable disease.

Since 2000, global efforts have been applied to reducing the burden of tuberculosis (TB) disease. Between 2000 and 2015, an estimated 49 million people were saved through TB diagnosis and treatment. The MDGs established targets to "halt and reverse" TB incidence by 2015, notably by halving TB prevalence and mortality rates by 2015 as compared with their levels in 1990.

Figure 1.8 shows global trends in TB prevalence rate from 1990 to 2015. The horizontal dashed lines represent the Stop TB Partnership targets of a 50% reduction in prevalence rate by 2015 as compared with 1990. Globally, TB prevalence dropped steeply, falling by 42% between 1990 and 2015. The MDG TB target of halving the prevalence rate was achieved in three WHO regions (America, South East Asia and the Western Pacific) and in nine high-burden countries (Brazil, Cambodia, China, Ethiopia, India, Myanmar, the Philippines, Uganda and Viet Nam). In 2015, the 87% of new TB cases occurred in the 30 TB high-burden countries: 61% of new TB cases occurred in Asia, followed by 26% in Africa. Six countries accounted for 60% of the new TB cases: India, Indonesia, China, Nigeria, Pakistan and South Africa.

Ending the TB epidemic by 2030 is therefore an urgent public health emergency and has been included among the health targets of the SDGs.

In 2015 there were 10.4 million new TB cases (including 1.2 million among HIV-positive people), of which 5.9 million were among men, 3.5 million among women and 1.0 million among children. Overall, 90% of cases were adults and 10% children.

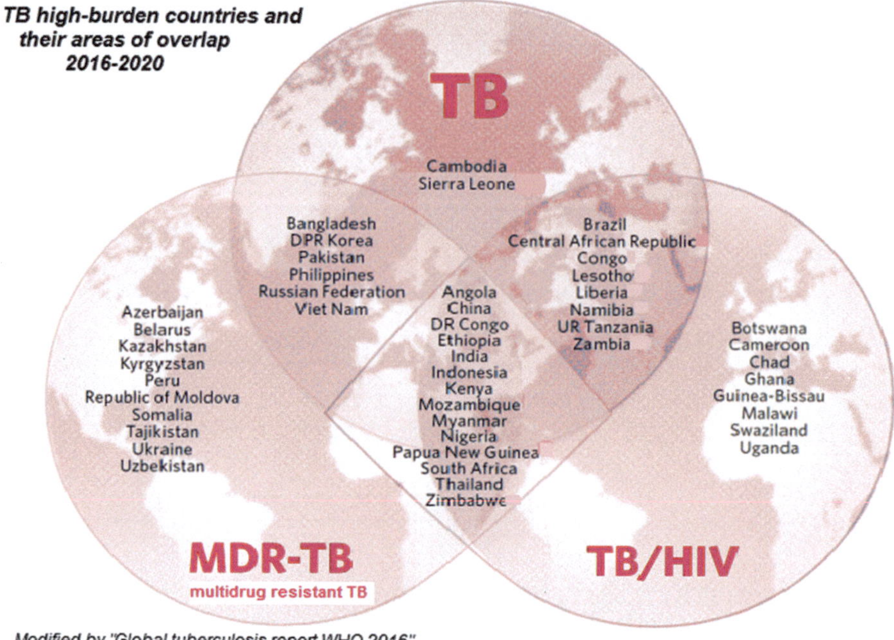

Fig. 1.9 TB high-burden countries and their areas of overlapping with HIV and MDR-TB

People infected with TB bacteria have a 10% lifetime risk of falling ill with TB. TB and HIV are a lethal combination: people living with HIV have compromised immune systems, so they have a much higher risk of falling ill (20–30 times more risk).

In 2015 there were 1.4 million TB deaths and an additional 0.4 million deaths resulting from TB disease among HIV-positive people. When anti-TB medicines are used inappropriately (incorrect prescription, poor-quality drugs, poor adherence to treatment), a drug resistance can occur. Multidrug-resistant tuberculosis (MDR-TB) is a form of TB caused by bacteria that do not respond to the first-line anti-TB drugs, thus making it necessary to use second-line drugs. However, second-line treatment options are limited and require extensive chemotherapy (up to 2 years of treatment) with medicines that are expensive and toxic. Figure 1.9 shows the overlap of TB, HIV and MDR-TB in TB high-burden countries. Over 95% of TB deaths occur in low- and middle-income countries.

1.4　Malaria: Epidemiological Perspective

Malaria is an acute febrile illness caused by *Plasmodium* parasites. The parasites are spread to people through the "malaria vectors", the infected female *Anopheles* mosquitoes. Two of the five species of *Plasmodium* (*P. falciparum* and *P. vivax*)

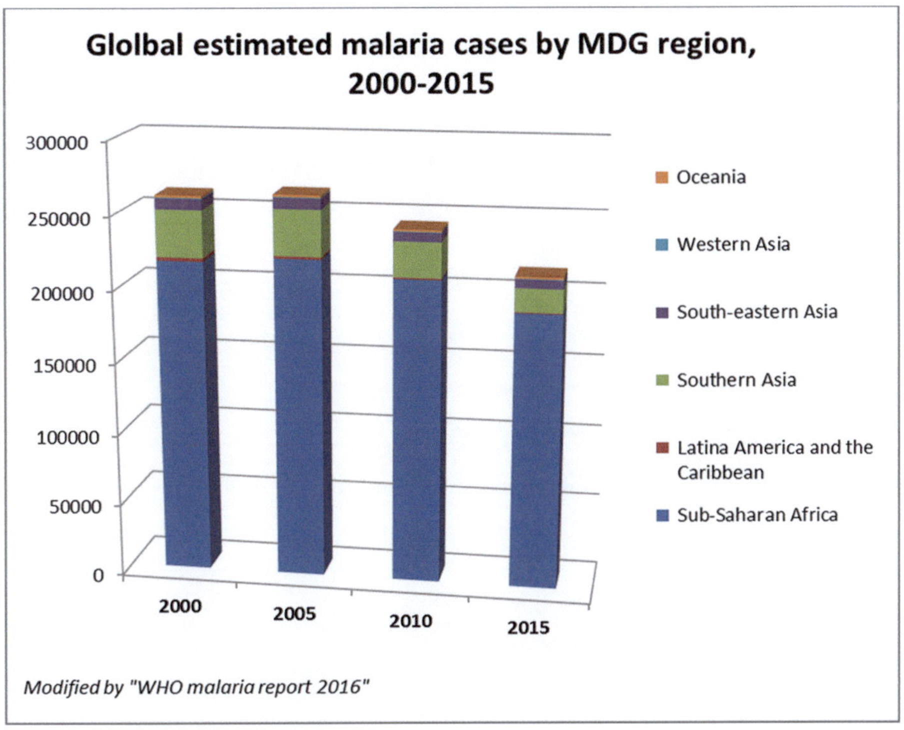

Fig. 1.10 Global TB prevalence rate

pose the greatest threat. According to the last *WHO World Malaria Report*, in 2015 there were globally 212 million cases of malaria and 429,000 malaria-related deaths. As you can see in Fig. 1.10, the sub-Saharan African region accounted for 90% of global cases of malaria, followed by the South East Asia region (7%).

P. falciparum is the most prevalent malaria parasite on the African continent, responsible for most malaria-related deaths globally. Figures 1.11 and 1.12 report the situation in sub-Saharan Africa: in the first picture, we can see the prevalence of *Plasmodium* parasite correlates with proportion of population infected; in the second one, we can see the number of people infected by malaria. In both figures, data are reported as age between 2 and 10 years compared with other ages. In fact, in those regions where the transmission of malaria is high, children (more especially under 5 years of age) are particularly susceptible to this infection: 70% of all malaria deaths occur in this age group. Between 2010 and 2015, the malaria mortality rate among children under 5 fell by nearly 35%. Nevertheless, malaria claims the life of one child every 2 minutes, remaining a major killer of children under 5 years.

MDG target of malaria included the halting of the disease by 2015 and the start of a reversal trend in the incidence of malaria and other major diseases. Globally MDGs for malaria have been met convincingly.

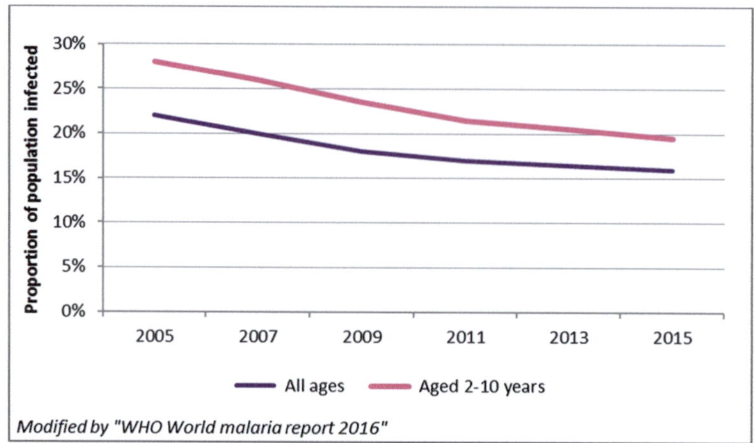

Fig. 1.11 Estimated parasite prevalence in sub-Saharan Africa, 2005–2015

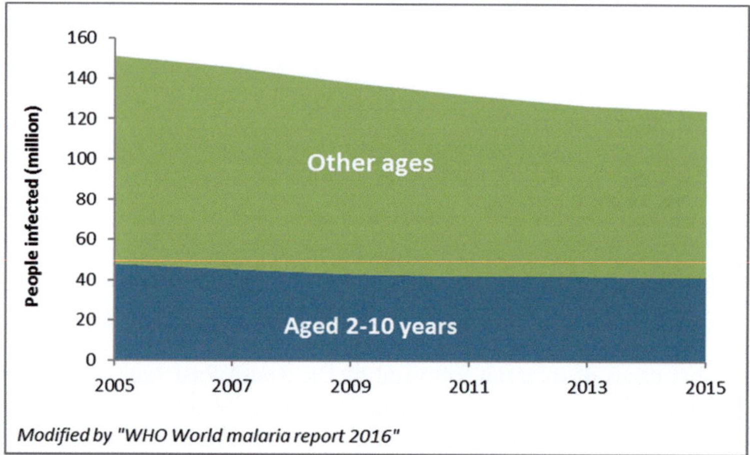

Fig. 1.12 Number of people infected by malaria in sub-Saharan Africa, 2000–2015

Figure 1.13 shows how this goal was achieved in African countries from 2000 to 2015. Despite impressive progress, the disease remains still concentrated in Africa, and most of the countries in sub-Saharan Africa have not met the specific target. Rates of decrease in malaria incidence in these countries between 2000 and 2015 (32%) lag behind the rates seen in other countries (54%). There is a strong need to rapidly accelerate the disease incidence reduction in these countries.

MDG Target on malaria incidence reduction in African countries, 2000-2015.

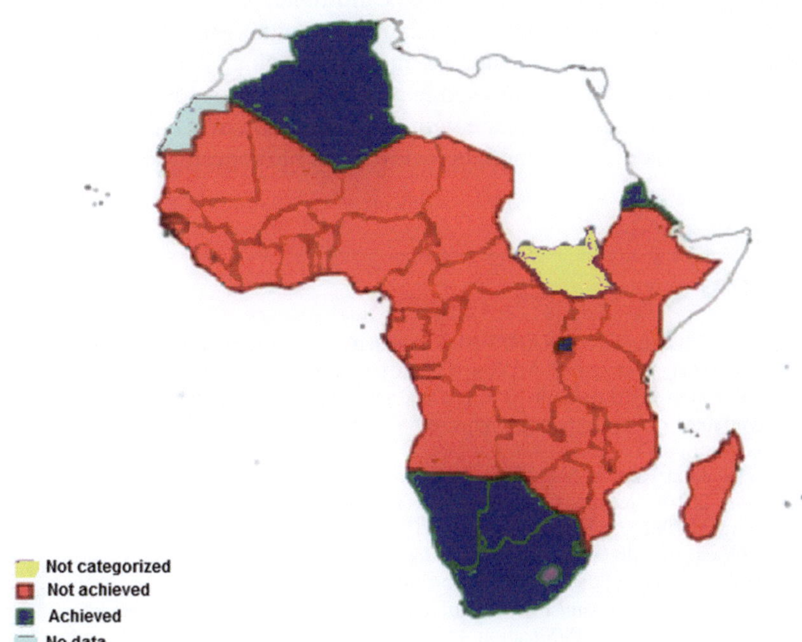

Modified by "Atlas of African Health Statistics 2016: Health situation analysis of the African Region. WHO 2016"

Fig. 1.13 MDG target on malaria incidence in Africa, 2000–2015

The WHO strategy to combat malaria sets ambitious but attainable goals for 2020:

1. Reducing malaria case incidence by at least 40%
2. Reducing malaria mortality rates by at least 40%
3. Eliminating malaria in at least ten countries
4. Preventing a resurgence of malaria in all countries that are malaria-free

There are three main ways to prevent and fight malaria:

- Control the vector, using insecticide-treated mosquito nets (ITNs) or indoor residual spraying (IRS), to block the parasite-mosquito-human circle.
- Chemoprevention to suppress the stage of blood infection in humans and prevent the onset of the disease; Case management, by enhancing prompt diagnosis and treatment with appropriate antimalarial medicines, to reduce the likelihood of progression to severe disease and death.

Malaria vaccines could be a strong weapon in the potential prevention of malaria disease and reduction of its transmission. Unfortunately, the complexity of the malaria parasite makes development of a malaria vaccine very challenging. There is currently no commercially available malaria vaccine, but over 20 vaccine constructs are currently being evaluated in clinical trials or in advanced preclinical tests. Recent progress has been made with the completion of a Phase 3 trial of the RTS,S/AS01 candidate vaccine and its review by the European Medicines Agency and WHO.

Bibliography

UNAIDS. Global AIDS update. UNAIDS 2016. Available online at: http://www.unaids.org/sites/default/files/media_asset/global-AIDS-update-2016_en.pdf

WHO. Progress report 2016 prevent HIV, test and treat all—WHO support for country impact. 2016. Available online at: http://apps.who.int/iris/bitstream/10665/251713/1/WHO-HIV-2016.24-eng.pdf

WHO. World Malaria Report 2016. World Health Organization 2016. Geneva: World Health Organization; 2016. Licence: CC BY-NC-SA 3.0 IGO. Available online at: http://apps.who.int/iris/bitstream/10665/252038/1/9789241511711-eng.pdf?ua=1

WHO/AFRO Library Cataloguing—in—Publication Data Atlas of African Health Statistics 2016: Health situation analysis of the African Region. WHO Regional Office for Africa, 2016. Available at: http://www.aho.afro.who.int/sites/default/files/publications/5266/Atlas-2016-en.pdf

WHO Library Cataloguing-in-Publication Data. Accelerating progress on HIV, tuberculosis, malaria, hepatitis and neglected tropical diseases. A new agenda for 2016–2030. World Health Organization 2015. Available online at: http://apps.who.int/iris/bitstream/10665/204419/1/9789241510134_eng.pdf?ua=1

WHO Library Cataloguing-in-Publication Data. Global Tuberculosis report 2016. World Health Organization 2016. Available online at: http://apps.who.int/iris/bitstream/10665/250441/1/9789241565394-eng.pdf?ua=1

World health statistics 2017: monitoring health for the SDGs, Sustainable Development Goals. Geneva: World Health Organization; 2017. Licence: CC BY-NC-SA 3.0 IGO. Available online at: http://www.who.int/gho/publications/world_health_statistics/2016/en/

Sandro Petrolati and Fabio Ferrari

2.1 The Incidence of Chronic Diseases in the World

In April 2017, the World Health Organisation reported that non-communicable diseases are the cause of death of 40 million people a year (around 70% of all deaths worldwide). The greatest number of deaths are caused by cardiovascular diseases (17.7 million), followed by cancer (8.8 million), respiratory diseases (3.9 million) and diabetes (1.6 million). What is even more alarming is that 87% of the deaths occur in countries with a medium-low-income.

In 2011 the growing importance of non-communicable diseases throughout the world led the UN to dedicate a session regarding healthcare for the second time in its history (the first time was on HIV/AIDS). Representatives from the national governments of the UN came together in New York to discuss non-communicable diseases and in the first paragraph of the final resolution (66/2 of 19th and 20th September 2011) of the UN General Assembly, these representatives:

1. Acknowledge that the global burden and threat of non-communicable diseases constitutes one of the major challenges for development in the twenty-first century, which undermines social and economic development throughout the world and threatens the achievement of internationally agreed development goals.

The transition from a greater incidence of death from nutritional and infectious diseases to death from chronic-degenerative or non-communicable diseases is called an epidemiologic transition [1].

S. Petrolati (✉)
San Camillo Hospital, Rome, Italy
e-mail: sandropetrolati@gmail.com

F. Ferrari
University of Rome 'La Sapienza', Rome, Italy
e-mail: fabioferrari84@yahoo.it

© Springer International Publishing AG, part of Springer Nature 2018
M. Bartolo, F. Ferrari (eds.), *Multidisciplinary Teleconsultation in Developing Countries*, TELe-Health, https://doi.org/10.1007/978-3-319-72763-9_2

This change is clear from a report in the Lancet in September 2016 [2], which shows a significant reduction in infectious diseases. Infant mortality is falling faster than expected, although the figures are still very high. Maternal mortality is decreasing, though it is still dramatic in 24 countries (with over 400 deaths every 1000 people). There is better control of malaria and of HIV/AIDS and a reduction of the incidence of diarrhoea, due to the overall improvement of public health and healthcare, assessed in terms of the quality of living environments, the indoor air quality and infant malnutrition. It has been calculated that by 2030 the number of deaths worldwide from non-communicable diseases will have increased to nearly at 52 million.

2.2 Chronic-Degenerative Diseases in Medium-Low-Income Countries

As mentioned above, 87% of the deaths from non-communicable diseases are recorded in medium-low-income countries. These diseases cause death at an earlier age than in countries with a high income, and in fact 29% of the total number of deaths occur before 60 years of age in medium-low-income countries, compared to 13% in countries with a high-income. It is estimated that the increase in the incidence of cancer in 2030, compared to in 2008, will be greater in countries with a low-income (82%) and in those with a medium-low-income (70%) than the increase expected in medium-high (58%)- and high (40%)-income countries.

The non-communicable disease epidemic has a specific impact on people who belong to the lowest social levels. Non-communicable diseases and poverty are closely connected. Poverty exposes people to behavioural risk factors that generate or worsen these pathologies, and the onset of the latter can, in turn, become a further element that fuels the downward spiral. The result is an increase in poverty, since people are less able to work and they also have more healthcare costs to cover.

The increase in risk factors in the populations of medium- and low-income countries is determined one hand by the greater life expectancy, but also and above all, it is the consequence of the rapid urbanisation of these populations. It has been seen that the "urbanised" populations of developing countries tend to consume more and more high-calorie, low-quality food, and there is also an increase in the consumption of alcohol and tobacco. The increase in the consumption of alcohol and tobacco in these populations is also a result of different marketing strategies, since there has been a drop in the consumption, in particular of tobacco, in higher-income countries, so companies have had to look for new markets. Urbanised populations also tend to adopt a sedentary lifestyle.

In sub-Saharan Africa, there has been an increase in non-communicable diseases including cardiovascular diseases, metabolic diseases like diabetes and obesity, and cancer (Fig. 2.1).

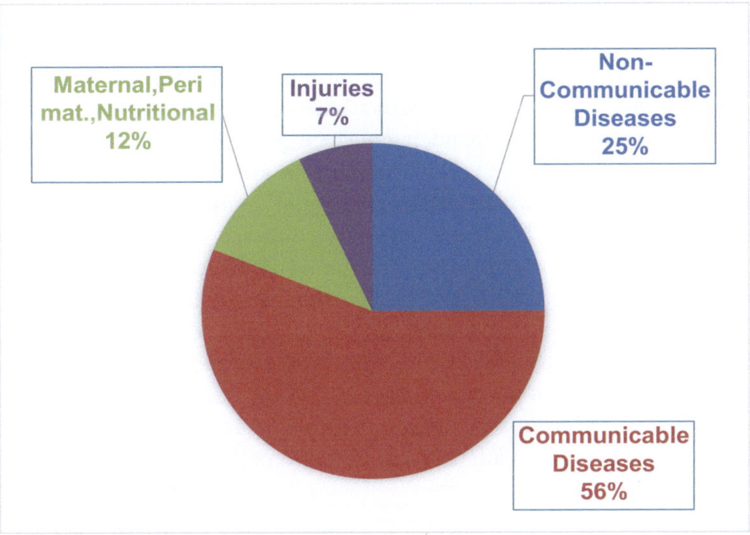

Fig. 2.1 Estimated causes of death in SSA 2004. Source: WHO. Global Burden of Disease. Projections of mortality and burden of disease, 2002–307. SSA, sub-Saharan Africa. 886 International Journal of Epidemiology 2011;40:885–901—Modified

2.3 Cardiovascular Diseases: A Model of Chronic-Degenerative Disease on the Increase in Countries in Sub-Saharan Africa

In sub-Saharan African countries, cardiovascular diseases are not epidemic; neither are they among the main causes of death. Nonetheless, since 1990 there has been a significant increase in deaths from cardiovascular diseases. Although the epidemiologic data is limited, the Global Burden Disease Study estimated that in these countries, cardiovascular diseases caused 8.8% of total deaths (38.3% of the deaths from NCD and 11% of the total deaths), with a total of 3.9% of years of life lost compared to life expectancy. Sub-Saharan Africa accounted for 5.5% of all the deaths from cardiovascular diseases in the world. The death rate from ischaemic heart disease in sub-Saharan Africa is the lowest in the world, with 2.3 deaths every 1000 inhabitants, compared to 18.9 of 1000 in Europe and 24.8 of 1000 in the United States. Nonetheless, its incidence is increasing, as shown by a WHO report [3]. In fact, in 2005 the number of deaths from ischaemic heart disease was 188,000 in men and 173,000 in women; by 2015 these figures were expected to have increased by 27% in men and by 25% in women and in 2030 by 70% in men and by 74% in women [4].

The increased incidence of ischaemic heart disease is directly related to the parallel increase in the traditional cardiovascular risk factors and the rapid changes related to a sedentary lifestyle, a different diet, economic development, urbanisation and also inevitably the increase in life expectancy [5].

In particular, the increase in urbanisation mentioned above causes significant changes in risk factors: in 1900 only around 5% of Africans were urbanised; in the 1950s, at the beginning of independence, urbanisation had risen to 14.7%; in 2000 this figure had reached 37.2%; and in 2015 it was around 45%.

In the ACE study [6], which includes African countries and the Middle East, 92% of the adults had at least one cardiovascular risk factor, and 53% of these people had three or more risk factors. The main risk factor among men is smoking and for women it is obesity. There is also a high incidence of risk factors among young people, which suggests the need to carry out early screening for the diagnosis and treatment of cardiovascular risk factors [6]. Moreover, in agreement with the Interheart African Study, a predictive model that includes five risk factors, that is, smoking, diabetes, hypertension, abdominal obesity and an altered apolipoprotein B/A1 ratio, identifies a population at an extremely high risk of heart attack (89%) [7].

This situation is also a consequence of the longer life expectancy, and the epidemiological data show that between 1990 and 2013, most of the cardiovascular diseases in sub-Saharan Africa were atrial fibrillation and peripheral arterial diseases.

Due to the increasing incidence of ischaemic heart disease, surgical and percutaneous approaches will have to be developed for the treatment of severe forms of coronary heart disease. With respect to this, a recent position paper by the South Africa Heart Association underlined the need to adapt the health systems of african countries to the rapid expansion of non-communicable diseases, including ischaemic heart disease [8]. With this in mind, in 2011 a clinical-scientific collaboration was set up between the Department of Cardiology in Nouakchott in Mauritania and the San Camillo Hospital in Rome (Italian Government programme project AID 9580/ICU/MRT). The aim is to teach surgical and percutaneous coronary revascularisation procedures, through continuous staff exchanges, with Italian haemodynamic doctors and heart surgeons spending time in Nouakchott.

Arterial hypertension is by far the most common risk factor for cardiovascular disease [9]. Africa has the highest incidence of hypertension: 46% of adults over 25 years of age, with a forecast for 2025 of 60%. The African Union declared arterial hypertension the most important healthcare challenge for Africa after HIV/AIDS, also considering its high social-economic impact. Despite the great difficulty in obtaining reliable data, it is estimated that 10–30% of the African population has arterial hypertension. In Western Africa the estimate is 30–40%. In 2000 it was estimated that 75–80 million Africans suffered from hypertension, double the number of people with HIV throughout the world. The estimate for 2015 was 150 million hypertensive people in Africa.

Unfortunately prevention, identification, treating and controlling arterial hypertension in sub-Saharan Africa take place randomly and are not easy to carry out in a widespread way. This is due to the absence of healthcare resources and facilities, the lack of adequate prevention strategies and the limited access to pharmacological therapies.

Rheumatic heart disease has almost completely disappeared in industrialised countries, whereas in developing countries it is still the main cause of cardio-vascular mortality and heart failure in children and young people. Most cases are found in sub-Saharan Africa, in the Pacific islands and in the aborigine populations of Australia. It is hard to obtain reliable epidemiologic data on the impact of rheumatic heart disease in developing countries, due to the difficulty of access to diagnosis. It is estimated that in these populations the prevalence varies between 5 and 80 cases per 100,000 inhabitants. In practically all cases, the diagnosis is made late, and when it is carried out, the only therapy left is surgery because at that point the valvular disease is advanced. Considering the costs and extremely limited possibilities of surgery, in most cases the disease evolves naturally. In many cases, valvular disease that is a consequence of rheumatic heart disease, in particular mitral stenosis, causes stroke even in young patients, because of the early onset of atrial fibrillation. Prevention, which in industrialised countries has almost eliminated rheumatic heart disease, includes prevention of the *Streptococcus* infection, treating relapses and early screening of subclinical forms of valvular disease. A study carried out by Elisabetta Rossi with an Italian team [10, 11] indicated a high prevalence of rheumatic heart disease (4%) among high school students. The study also showed the importance of early echocardiographic screening and rheumatic fever prevention campaigns.

Atrial fibrillation is present in sub-Saharan African countries at a far younger age than in countries with a medium-high income for two main reasons: the high incidence of valvular disease, in particular rheumatic mitral stenosis, and the large number of hypertensive patients, also at a young age. It is more prevalent in men, but mortality is higher in women.

The number of deaths from atrial fibrillation increased by 196% in 2013 compared to 1990. Atrial fibrillation, as it is known, involves a high risk of thrombo-embolic complications, particularly stroke, especially when there is an underlying rheumatic valvular heart disease.

Heart failure is a major cause of death and disability in sub-Saharan Africa. A recent global review of the aetiology, epidemiology and clinical aspects of heart failure in sub-Saharan Africa, carried out by Bloomfield et al., showed that this syndrome also has mainly "non-ischaemic" causes. In most cases it is a question of hypertensive heart disease, rheumatic heart disease and cardiomyopathies. THESUS-HF, the first heart failure registry in Africa, came to the same conclusion.

Nonetheless, it has been pointed out that although atherosclerotic cardiovascular disease (in which diabetes plays an important role) is apparently rarer, with the limited data available, it is not possible to have an accurate picture of the extent of the atherosclerotic heart disease.

Peripheral artery disease has been one of the cardiovascular diseases with the highest increase in sub-Saharan Africa since 1990 and, above all, with high rates of increase in the population under 55 years of age. This indicates a greater exposure to risk factors like smoking, diabetes, hypertension and hypercholesterolemia, at a relatively young age.

The high incidence of *cerebrovascular disease* in this part of Africa represents a serious healthcare problem: death from stroke almost doubled between 1990 and 2013. Haemorrhagic stroke is more frequent than ischaemic stroke: this inversion compared to other parts of the world is explained by the lower incidence in the population of the forms caused by atherosclerosis and a higher presence, as mentioned above, of arterial hypertension.

It is important to underline that the knowledge of the relationship between socioeconomic and cardiovascular risk factors at the time of the epidemiological transition is a crucial step in order to develop scientific-based guidelines for national and global policies and priorities.

2.4   Metabolic Diseases: Diabetes in Sub-Saharan Africa

Diabetes has actually become an epidemic disease; according to the data collected by the IDF (International Diabetes Federation), the number of adult deaths caused by diabetes is significantly higher than those caused by the most widespread pathologies in Africa, like HIV/AIDS, TB and malaria, put together [12].

Diabetes	HIV/AIDS	Tuberculosis	Malaria
4 million (2017) IFD	1.5 million (2013) WHO	1.5 million (2013) WHO	0.6 million (2013) WHO

Source: Diabetes Atlas (IDF 2017), WHO 2013

In 2015 there were around 468 million people living in sub-Saharan Africa, with a prevalence of diabetes of around 3.3%, that is, around 15 million people. According to estimates, the number of people with diabetes is expected to increase by 162.5% by 2045. Most of the people with diabetes live in urban areas (58%). In this epidemic there are far fewer cases of diabetes type 1 under the age of 20, the prevalence is around 50,600 cases.

The prevalence varies considerably from country to country, and this reflects the rapid social-economic changes in society. The highest prevalence is reported in Reunion (15.4%), followed by the Seychelles (12.1%), Gabon (10.7%) and Zimbabwe (9.7%). Some of the countries with the highest populations have the largest number of people with diabetes: Nigeria (3.9 million), South Africa (2.6 million), Ethiopia (1.9 million) and the Republic of Tanzania (1.7 million) [13].

A study carried out in 2009 estimated that the overall economic impact of diabetes in sub-Saharan Africa in 2000 was around $68 billion, the equivalent of $8800 per person with diabetes [14].

The 2017 IDF report calculated that USD3.3 billion (ID 6.7 billion) was spent on healthcare by people with diabetes, and this is the lowest from all seven IDF regions, representing less than 1% of the total spent worldwide, despite the region being home to 3% of people with diabetes. The projection is that the amount spent by people with diabetes will double by 2045, reaching USD6.0 billion [11].

It is also estimated that over two thirds (66%) of the people with diabetes are undiagnosed [15].

In 2015, in the countries in sub-Saharan Africa, over 320,000 deaths were attributed to diabetes, and 79% of these people were under 60 years old, which is a negative record compared to all the other regions analysed. The death rate for women is 1.7 times greater than that for men, which is also likely to be due to the greater risk for men of dying from other causes (201,00000 women compared to 120,000 men in 2015) [16].

The WHO "Global Action Plan for the Prevention and Control of Non-communicable Diseases 2013–2020" includes the following among a series of actions:

1. Increasing the level of prevention by strengthening international cooperation.
2. Reduce the changeable risk factors for non-communicable diseases and the underlying social determining factors.

The resolution adopted by the World Health Assembly in Geneva in 2013 underlines the need to commit "to strengthen health systems towards the provision of equitable, universal health coverage and promote affordable access to prevention, treatment, care and support related to non-communicable diseases, especially cancer, cardiovascular diseases, chronic respiratory diseases and diabetes, and commits to establish or strengthen multisectoral national policies for the prevention and control of non-communicable diseases".

References

1. Yusuf S, Reddy S, Ounpuu S, Anand S. Global burden of cardiovascular diseases: part I: general considerations, the epidemiologic transition, risk factors, and impact of urbanization. Circulation. 2001;104:2746–53.
2. Measuring the health-related Sustainable Development Goals in 188 countries: a baseline analysis from the Global Burden of Disease Study 2015 (GBD).
3. World Health Organization. WHO Report 2006: working together for health.
4. World Health Organization. http://www.who.int/healthinfo/statistics/bod_deathbyregion.xls. Accessed 28 December 2011.
5. Dalal S. Int J Epidemiol. 2011;40:885–901.
6. Alsheikh-Ali AA, Omar MI, Raal FJ, Rashed W, Hamoui O, Kane A, Alami M, Abreu P, Mashhoud WM. Cardiovascular risk factor burden in Africa and the Middle East: the Africa Middle East Cardiovascular Epidemiological (ACE) study. PLoS One. 2014;9:e102830.
7. Steyn K, Sliwa K, Hawken S, Commerford P, Onen C, Damasceno A, et al. INTERHEART Investigators in Africa. Risk factors associated with myocardial infarction in Africa: the INTERHEART Africa study. Circulation. 2005;112:3554–61.
8. Sliwa K, Zühlke L, Kleinloog R, Doubell A, Ebrahim I, Essop M, et al. Cardiology-cardiothoracic subspeciality training in South Africa: a position paper of the South Africa Heart Association. Cardiovasc J Afr. 2016;27:188–93.

9. Cappuccio FP, Miller MA. Cardiovascular disease and hypertension in sub-Saharan Africa: burden, risk and interventions. Intern Emerg Med. 2016;11:299–305.
10. Rossi E, Felici AR, Banteyrga L. Subclinical rheumatic heart disease in an Eritrean high-school population detected by echocardiography. J Heart Valve Dis. 2014 Mar;23(2):235–9.
11. IDF – International Diabetes Federation. Atlas of Diabetes, 8th ed; 2017.
12. WHO – World Health Organization. Global Report on Diabetes; 2016.
13. Readmission and death after an acute heart failure event: predictors and outcomes in sub-Saharan Africa: results from the THESUS-HF registry.
14. http://www.who.int/neglected_diseases/WHA_66_seventh_day_resolution_adopted/en/
15. ibidem.
16. Ibidem.

References with no reference to the text

17. WHO Fact sheet Updated April 2017.
18. WHO Library Data Global status report on noncommunicable diseases 2014. World Health Organization. ISBN 978 92 4 156485 4 – NLM classification: WT 500 – © World Health Organization 2014.
19. Aminde LN, Dzudie A, Andre Pascal Kengne. Prevalent diabetes mellitus in patients with heart failure and disease determinants in sub-Saharan Africans having diabetes with heart failure: a protocol for a systematic review and meta-analysis. BMJ Open. 2016; 6(2):e010097.
20. George A Mensah, MD, Uchechukwu KA Sampson, MD, Gregory A Roth, MD, Mohammed H Forouzanfar, MD, Mohsen Naghavi, MD, Christopher JL Murray, MD, Andrew E Moran, MD, Valery L Feigin, MD. Mortality from cardiovascular diseases in sub-Saharan Africa, 1990–2013: a systematic analysis of data from the Global Burden of Disease Study 2013. Cardiovasc J Afr. 2015 Mar–Apr; 26(2 H3Africa Suppl):S6–S10.
21. "Measuring the health-related Sustainable Development Goals in 188 countries: a baseline analysis from the Global Burden of Disease Study 2015(GBD)", Lancet sett.2016.
22. Moran A, Forouzanfar M, Sampson U, Chugh S, Feigin V, Mensah G. The epidemiology of cardiovascular diseases in sub-Saharan Africa: the Global Burden of Diseases, Injuries and Risk Factors 2010 Study. Prog Cardiovasc Dis. 2013 Nov–Dec;56(3):234–9. doi: https://doi.org/10.1016/j.pcad.2013.09.019. Epub 2013 Sep 28.
23. Anastase Dzudie, MD, PhD, FESC, Abdoul Kane, MD, Euloge Kramoh, MD, Jean-Baptiste Anzouan-Kacou, MD, Jean Marie, Damourou, MD, Lucien Allawaye, MD, Jolis Nzisabira, MD, Latif Mousse, MD, Dadier Balde, MD, Ouane Nouhom, MD, Jean, Louis Nkoa,, MD, Kimbally Kaki, MD, Armel Djomou, MD, Alain Menanga, MD, Samuel Kingue, MD, Christ Nadege Nganou, MD, Liliane Mfeukeu Kuate, MD, Jean Bruno Mipinda, MD, Lucie Nebie, MD, and Serigne Abdou Ba MD. Development of the roadmap for reducing cardiovascular morbidity and mortality through the detection, treatment and control of hypertension in Africa: report of a working group of the PAS CAR Hypertension Task Force. Cardiovasc J Afr. 2016 May–Jun; 27(3): 200–2.

Part II
DREAM 2.0

From DREAM to DREAM 2.0: An African Model

3

Maria Cristina Marazzi

3.1   The Origin of the DREAM Programme

After working in Mozambique for peace and reaching an agreement that was signed in October 1992 [1], the Community of Sant'Egidio became aware of the increasing drama of AIDS in the country. The war was over, but many people were still dying in Mozambique. It was the end of the 1990s and the scientific world, the local governments and the World Health Organization itself identified prevention as the only possible way to counter HIV/AIDS in Africa [2–5].

The failure of that decision, which was apparently inexpensive but not very scientific, was rapidly made evident by the growing number of deaths throughout Africa, by the alarming reduction in life expectancy in the countries affected and, above all, by the lack of control of the infection. Despite the health education campaigns, there was an increase in the stigma; sick people were rejected and often their families too.

Starting from the clearly wrong healthcare decisions that had been made up to then, a group of doctors who also carried out research, from the Community of Sant'Egidio, suggested that prevention had to be combined with therapy, as a natural complement in reducing the number of new infections. In 1999, with this belief, backed by strong scientific evidence [6, 7], advocacy activities were started in order to persuade the Mozambican Government to make the use of the therapy in the country legal and to allow the antiretroviral drugs commonly used in the Western world to be imported.

At the beginning the local authorities had only doubts and fears. An attempt to do something like this had recently failed in South Africa [8, 9] leaving behind it serious social problems. What guarantees could the Community of Sant'Egidio

M. C. Marazzi (✉)
Department of Humanities – Communication, Education, Psychology, LUMSA University, Rome, Italy
e-mail: marazzi@lumsa.it

© Springer International Publishing AG, part of Springer Nature 2018
M. Bartolo, F. Ferrari (eds.), *Multidisciplinary Teleconsultation in Developing Countries*, TELe-Health, https://doi.org/10.1007/978-3-319-72763-9_3

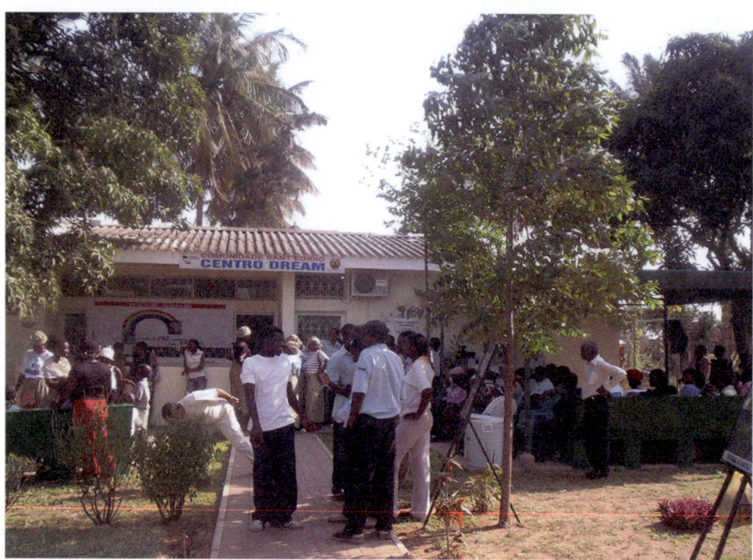

Fig. 3.1 Machava: first DREAM health centre. Suburbs of Maputo - Mozambique

provide, at least in the short term, from a point of view of continuity and sustainability? Besides, who on earth would fund and support a project that had been rejected from the start and was not even taken into consideration by the relevant national and international organisations? This is how negotiations with the Mozambican authorities began, and at the same time a project, to make people more aware of the AIDS problem through a homecare service in the outskirts of Maputo for HIV+ patients suffering from various opportunistic infections.

The first authorisation to import antiretroviral drugs in Mozambique arrived after 2 years of work and negotiations, also thanks to the excellent work carried out by the Community of Sant'Egidio during the peace talks.

So in 2002 the first centre was set up, at the tuberculosis reference hospital in the outskirts of Maputo, for the prevention and treatment of AIDS and the fight against malnutrition. It was set up there so that it would not be too noticeable, would not be easy to get to and would not interfere with the country's healthcare programmes (Fig. 3.1).

This first treatment centre on the outskirts of Maputo soon became a reference centre and a lifesaver for many sick people (Fig. 3.2).

This is how DREAM started, with its ethical and scientific principles, convinced that the therapy had to depend on the patients' clinical evidence alone and not on their geographical location.

The general idea throughout the international scientific community, that Africa had to be left with its 30 million people with AIDS and no therapy, was unacceptable [10].

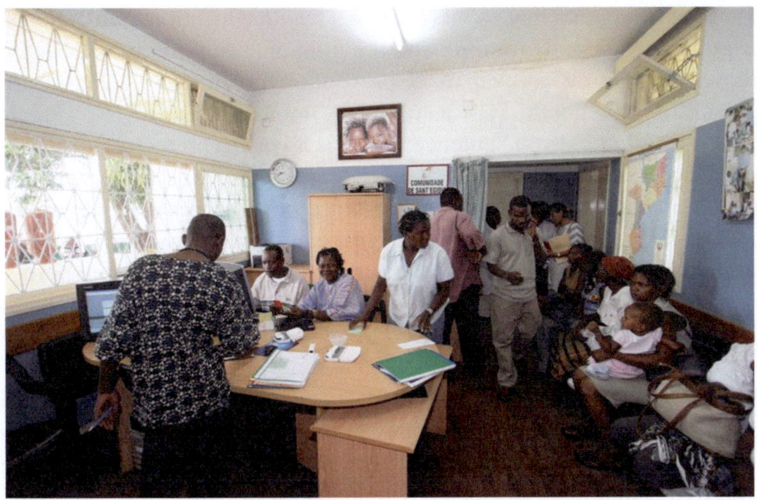

Fig. 3.2 DREAM health center in Mozambique

In a few years, this figure would have risen, leading to inevitable deaths, the number of which would have been comparable to a genocide. It was therefore necessary to work to show that the antiretroviral therapy was possible with the same quality, excellence and effectiveness as was achieved in Western countries.

At first, only a few members of the international scientific world agreed with DREAM's pioneering commitment to treating AIDS in Africa and were aware that treatment programmes could also really be introduced to Africa. One of these was the president of the International AIDS Society, Joep Lange, who at the International AIDS Conference in Barcelona in 2002 said: "If we can get cold Coca-Cola & beer to every remote corner of Africa, it shouldn't be impossible to do the same with drugs" [11].

Gradually and faced with the evidence, the irremovable convictions of the international organisations, which at the beginning had not even taken into consideration the hypothesis of introducing the therapy to developing countries, began to waver [12].

This is what Stephen Lewis, the UN Special Envoy for HIV/AIDS in Africa, said on December 1, 2005, on the occasion of the World AIDS Day: "Why do we tolerate one regimen for Africa (second-rate) and another for the rich nations (first rate)? Why do we tolerate the carnage of African children, and save the life of every western child? (...) It leaves the mind reeling to think of the millions of children who should be alive and aren't alive, simply because the world imposes such an obscene division between rich and poor" [13].

DREAM was set up precisely to fight AIDS in Africa, in order to make not only the antiretroviral therapy accessible but mother-to-child prevention as well and also to support everything that makes this possible: health education, nutritional support, advanced diagnostics, staff training and the fight against opportunistic infections.

Moreover the therapy has even made prevention more effective. People today are no longer afraid of taking the HIV test; finding out that you are HIV+ is no longer a question of receiving a death sentence, but it is a way to protect yourself and other people. The women who were not taken into considered and those who were then were treated as outcasts because of the disease have become the centre of a new awareness and represent the possibility to react and start living a new life—and also the men, their neighbours and the whole village. The children who are born healthy, thanks to the DREAM mother-to-child prevention programme, will not be added to the millions of orphans or be destined to live in the streets or in families with only grandparents and children and no middle generations.

Today 16 years later, it is wonderful to see how successful the DREAM programme has been, how fast it has spread in Africa and the influence it has had in changing the attitude of governments and international organisations regarding the antiretroviral therapies (ref). The results achieved, which are illustrated in the next chapters, have also been very important for the World Health Organisation in modifying the therapeutic protocols for Africa [14].

3.2   DREAM 2.0: The Growth of the Programme

DREAM's work over the years has shown the enormous impact that investing in treating AIDS has had on the healthcare systems. Specifically trained staff, new infrastructures, the organisation of the services and treatment models led to changes in the national guidelines and created a typically African way of managing the treatment, which is completely new and can also be adopted for other diseases. Today with the therapy, the HIV+ patients achieve a good quality of life and longer life expectancy, so they have to deal with other diseases. This unexpected life of so many sick people has therefore presented new demands that could not be ignored.

So in 2015 DREAM changed from Drug Resource Enhancement against AIDS and Malnutrition to DREAM 2.0 Disease Relief through Excellent and Advanced Means [15]. This is a model that no longer only fights HIV/AIDS but also other infectious diseases and many chronic pathologies which, applying the best diagnostic and therapeutic protocols in the world, has been adapted so it can work in Africa. So DREAM 2.0 gives a considerable contribution to the continent.

In fact over the years, its holistic approach to the patients' health has led DREAM to use instruments and skills for the many varied problems and pathologies that AIDS patients and in general many African patients suffer from. DREAM therefore started concentrating on the most frequently found diseases in Africa: anaemia, hepatitis, tuberculosis, malaria, some types of cancer and then the pathologies related to the Africans' increased life expectancy, like cardiovascular pathologies, hypertension and metabolic diseases including diabetes mellitus.

These pathologies are treated and monitored also thanks to the multidisciplinary teleconsultation service, which is a new way of monitoring every single person's overall health. This takes place through access to excellent diagnostics and advice regarding therapy. The next chapter of the book will describe this service and how it works.

One of the secrets to DREAM's success is the fact that from the very beginning, it invested in excellence in terms of technology, diagnostics and computerization. This was a difficult decision and not one that everybody understood. What was the point of taking computers to places where even the electric power supply was a problem?

This book describes how these difficulties and certain prejudices were overcome, and it is also the story of the success of technology. Technology is always at the service of man.

In fact over the years, the DREAM programme has created a software designed specifically for Africans; it has been translated into several languages and has been adopted as the national platform by the Ministry of Health of some countries in Africa.

The software was initially designed to manage the patient's clinical progress, and it later developed several areas concerning the person as a whole, their family and their social context. It keeps track of the social activities in the villages, the homecare service, the pharmacy and the communications with the laboratory, and through the teleconsultation service, it is also in contact with hundreds of Italian professionals and some from other European countries. This is a holistic software for a holistic treatment programme, which has helped DREAM's patients achieve excellent adherence to the treatment.

Using such complete software is also something extremely gratifying for the local health staff. This is also very important, but ICT experts do not often take this aspect into account.

Today with this software, it is possible to keep track of the clinical condition of 350,000 patients in 47 DREAM centres in 11 sub-Saharan African countries. The next chapters explain the software in detail.

Before looking at the technical and scientific aspects of the software, it is important to remember that one crucial key to the effectiveness of DREAM programme is the fact that it is based on spiritual and human values. It can be described as a healthcare programme with a soul. Its perspective is closely linked to that of the Community of Sant'Egidio: to work for a new world, feeling the responsibility to bravely and patiently build new paths that are a concrete and feasible answer to an enormous problem that the international organisations and Africa itself did not know how to solve. It is this soul that has made it possible to create unexpected synergies and become a model that can be replicated, with no jealousy issues concerning copyright, in the persistent pursuit of guaranteeing the same high-quality standards everywhere, which represents a guarantee of success.

References

1. Morozzo della Rocca R. Limes rivista Italiana di geopolitica. Sant'Egidio: la via romana alla pace, 1993. Available on http://www.limesonline.com/cartaceo/santegidio-la-via-romana-alla-pace?prv=true
2. Adler MW. Antiretrovirals for developing world. The Lancet. January 24, 1998; 351.
3. Hirshel B. Progress and problems in the fight against AIDS. N Engl J Med. 1998;338 (13):906–8.
4. Brown D. With fanfare, global aids conference gets underway in Vancouver. Washington Post, 8/07/1996.
5. Zeit P. Lessons from South Africa's experience of HIV/AIDS. The Lancet. 2007;370 (9581):19–20.
6. Royce RA, et al. Sexual transmission of HIV. N Engl J Med. 1997;336(15):1072–8.
7. Quinn TC, et al. for the Rakai Project Study Group. Viral load and heterosexual transmission of human immunodeficiency virus type 1. N Engl J Med 2000;342:921–9.
8. Simelela NP, et al. A brief history of South Africa's response to AIDS. S Afr Med J. 2014;104 (3 Suppl 1):249–51.
9. Furman K. Mbeki's AIDS denialism: Thabo Mbeki's support of dissident HIV/AIDS scientists is a cautionary tale for policy makers dealing with competing sets of evidence. Think Africa Press; 17 November 2011.
10. UNAIDS. Report on the global HIV/AIDS epidemic. Luglio 2002.
11. Lange J. Talking at the closing ceremony of the 14th IAS Conference. Barcellona Luglio; 2002.
12. WHO. Comunità di Sant'Egidio DREAM. An integrated faith-based initiative to treat HIV/AIDS in Mozambique. Case Study. Perspectives and Practice in Antiretroviral Treatment, Ginevra; 2005.
13. Statement by Stephen Lewis, UN Special Envoy for HIV/AIDS in Africa, on World AIDS Day, December 1, 2005.
14. "Adult Guideline Development Group" and "External Peer Reviewers" guideline WHO treatment HAART June 2003. WHO, Consolidated guidelines on the use of Antiretroviral drugs for treating and preventing HIV infection. Recommendations for a public health approach, Ginevra; 2013.
15. I sogni crescono: DREAM 2.0 ovvero Disease Relief through Excellent and Advanced Means 25 giugno 2015. Available on http://dream.santegidio.org/2015/06/25/i-sogni-crescono-dream-2-0-ovvero-disease-relief-through-excellent-and-advanced-means/

The DREAM Management Software

4

Marco Peroni and Flavio Ismael

A chapter describing the software used in the DREAM programme centres in Africa gives us an observation window, not only so we can understand the level of technology used in every healthcare centre, but also so we can have an overall view of how the centres, the organisation of the workflows and the activities of every single member of staff are organised.

The idea of using a simple database for managing and storing the patients' data goes back to 2002. At that time Microsoft had just released the first version of Windows XP and most PCs were still using Windows 98 or 2000. In Africa even an ordinary PC was something rare, especially in healthcare. The internet connection was only for a few, actually a very few people, and almost all the PCs were stand-alone PCs. Nobody expected us to decide to invest in technology.

Many people thought that the idea of introducing the same level of clinical treatment and technology that was used in the wealthy countries in the north of the world was bound to fail. An intervention that was too elaborate, both from a healthcare point of view and also because of the technologies used, was considered unrealistic, difficult to implement and even less sustainable or scalable on a national level. Therefore a simplified and minimalist intervention seemed to offer a greater guarantee of success and sustainability.

It was easy to justify people's wariness, because of the technological aspects, the concrete problems caused by the digital divide, the lack of stable electric power, above all in rural areas, and the lack of a company network and local staff with the necessary know-how to offer the necessary maintenance.

M. Peroni (✉)
'DREAM Program', Community of Sant'Egidio, Rome, Italy
e-mail: marcoperoni@hotmail.com

F. Ismael
'DREAM Program', Maputo, Mozambique
e-mail: flavioismael@dream.org.mz

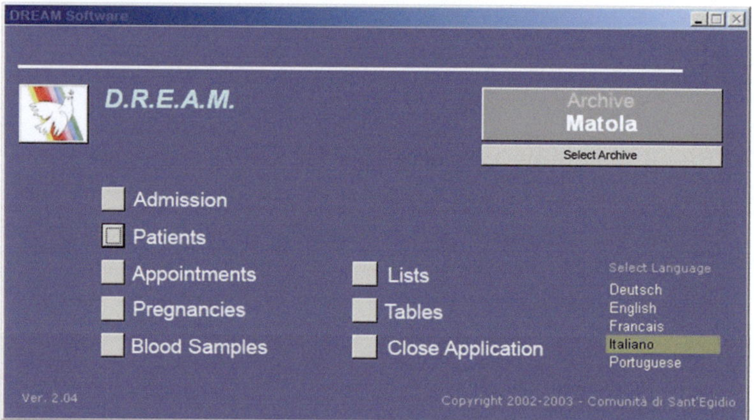

Fig. 4.1 Screenshot DREAM® Software (Authorised by ICT DREAM 2017)

Therefore in order to computerise the DREAM programme, it was not enough to provide software and a computer; there had to be an investment in infrastructures, training and constant support for the local staff.

We reacted to other people's resigned realism when faced with objective problems, with a high-level model, bearing in mind that we had to offer all round, long-term support. ICT, the building work, plumbing and electricity systems (see Chap. 14) were all dealt with as an integral part of the programme itself and constituted complex but well-defined know-how, which is essential for the replication of the DREAM model. Alongside healthcare training, there was technological training, in order to have professionals who could provide the maintenance and manage the scaling up of the infrastructures, the technological hardware and the computer systems. This training was not intended to consist of courses alone, but above all it provided everyday support, for continuous training. A large investment was therefore made in telecommunications, with an internet connection in every healthcare centre. This made it easier to contact the healthcare support network but also the technological help desk: it was a real cultural revolution. The staff of the DREAM centres use the computers perfectly competently and efficiently every day, and they maintain national and also international relations for training and support. This represents an important change in the way the work is carried out, and it has had a positive effect, not only within the programme itself, but it has also proved to be the most practical way to contribute to overcome the phenomenon of the digital divide and not be resigned to accepting it as a fact.

The technological challenge started in March 2002, when the doctors and nurses were sitting around a table and we presented the first version of the software with some portable PCs. At that time the software was very basic and used forms created with Microsoft Access (Fig. 4.1).

4.1   DREAM Software

That first software prototype only managed the patients' personal details and a simple clinical record. Today, after many other versions and after adopting new technological solutions, we have version 5 of DREAM Software. This software manages two modules: DREAMCen for managing the clinical centres and DREAMLab for managing the molecular biology and analysis laboratories.

Today's software has been made using the .NET Framework in C# and is able to connect to several database engines. At the moment DREAM Software manages 47 health centres and 25 laboratories and is supported by ICT staff, based in Rome, consisting of one director, 3 developers and 2 systems engineers, as well as the local experts in every country where there is the DREAM programme.

The DREAMCen module, which initially could be defined as an electronic medical record (EMR) software, today has become a complete point of care software [1], which is able to support the DREAM programme as a whole and not only the management of the patients' clinical diary and their personal details. This new software offers instruments that can optimise the flow and care of the patients and encourage and monitor their adherence to the treatments and their retention. DREAMCen also manages the movements of the drugs and of the healthcare materials, the food storerooms, the homecare assistance activities, the appointments schedules and the planning of the centres' everyday work.

It is important to mention that the software was not developed separately from the healthcare staff's work but with close collaboration on the field, in order to be able to identify which functions and priorities to develop, from the point of view of the final users. The healthcare staff were actively involved in every phase of the planning and implementation of the software [2].

The observations gathered on the field and the requests to implement new functions or to correct the users' errors were collected in a tool online [3] in order to define the priorities and to assign the development and verification tasks to the developers, in a relationship that has continued over the years and has made it possible for the software to continue to evolve up to today.

In-house development, with the developers in close contact with the coordinators of the healthcare programme, has made it possible to optimise the integration between the model of intervention, the software training and the development of software support instruments. It has therefore been possible to produce a model which, despite its complexity, is replicable and also successful in terms of the benefits that it gives the final users.

Describing all the functions of the DREAM software would require a separate book. Here we describe just a few specific issues that led us to develop a decisively "African" software.

4.2 Social Data Management

First of all, in line with DREAM programme's holistic approach to patients, the software integrates healthcare and social information, so that it is possible to have an overall view of the person that is not limited to their clinical condition. Knowing, for example, the distance and the time required for the patient to reach the healthcare centre, or how many people there are in their family, helps fine-tune the assistance and provides a solution if they have trouble following their treatment plan.

The user management system in the software makes it possible to decide what information and functions can be visualised and modified by the various users in a detailed and flexible way, so that it can be adapted to the different contexts in which it is used. This way it is possible to decide, for every user, whether the various functions are enabled or disabled and whether or not to display certain information.

In fact some sections of the software are used by non-healthcare staff, who are essential for the development of the programme, like the testimonials who are involved in awareness raising and who work on the homecare programme offering support for the treatments. These people have a particular user profile and can only access the information they need to carry out their work and no more than that, to guarantee the patients' privacy.

Looking at the programme's home page (Fig. 4.2), one can see the various sections organised in panels, each of which is real plug-in software that can be

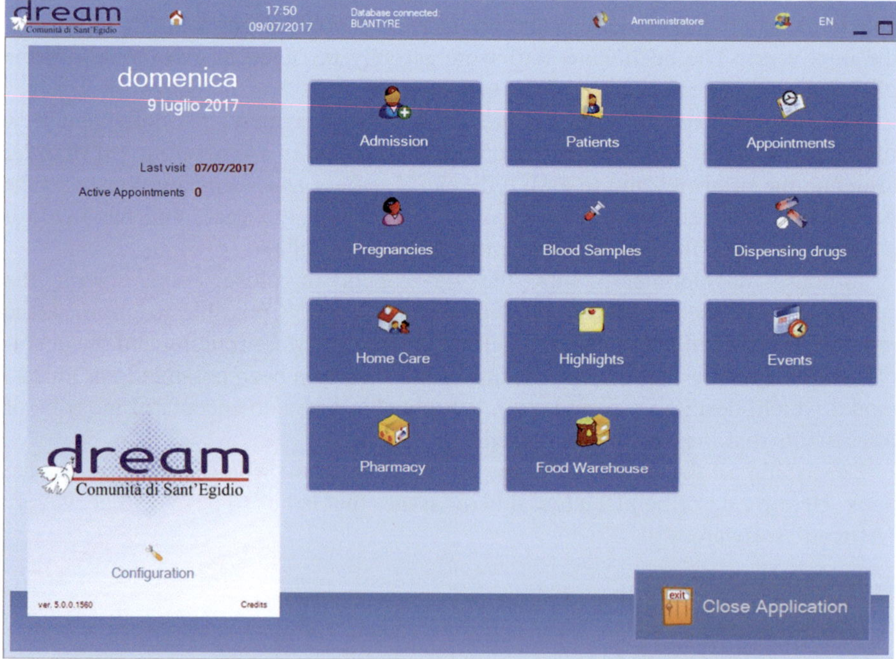

Fig. 4.2 The software's home page. Screenshot DREAM® Software (Authorised by ICT DREAM 2017)

enabled or not according to each centre's operational requirements. In fact all the software has been designed with a modular architecture around a central nucleus, so that new operational units can be added without losing the connections between the various modules. In addition to this structural flexibility, it is also possible to personalise a practically infinite number of variables and clinical indictors so that new therapeutic protocols can easily be implemented. The reports and analysis sections can also be personalised according to the requests of the various national health systems.

4.3   Managing and Monitoring the Appointments

The management of the appointment schedules is a fundamental aspect of the management of the centre and also of the clinical protocols. The software helps identify the best time to give a patient an appointment, taking into consideration their clinical needs, but also the amount of work the healthcare centre has on any given day. Whether the patient goes to their appointment on the right day or not contributes to the assessment of their adherence to the treatment, while a system that checks difficult situations, which is also integrated in this system, helps identify and check the situations where there is a risk that the patient might abandon the therapy.

The information can always be visualised from two main perspectives: starting with the patient or else with the overall management of the healthcare centre. From a general point of view, for example, the appointments can be planned in such a way as to balance the number of appointments made over several days and organise the daily activities better. On the other hand, from the patient's point of view, as can be seen in Fig. 4.3, it is possible to check the number and percentage of appointments that the patient went to, if they went on the right day or if they missed any altogether. This is useful for evaluating the patient's adherence to the therapy and if the adherence is found to be inadequate, for offering counselling in order to try and solve the problems that make adherence difficult.

4.4   Dispensing Drugs

The software makes it possible to perform a detailed check on the appointment for dispensing the drugs. This is particularly useful for the AIDS treatment, since the therapy must not be interrupted because of the risk of creating drug resistances which lead to a worsening of the patients' clinical condition.

It is important to point out that when the patients go to the centre's pharmacy on the day of the appointment, they are easily recognised because they have an identification number, and then using a real electronic prescription, they receive the drugs prescribed for the specified period. The software helps calculate the quantities required, and for the medication that has a pill count, like the

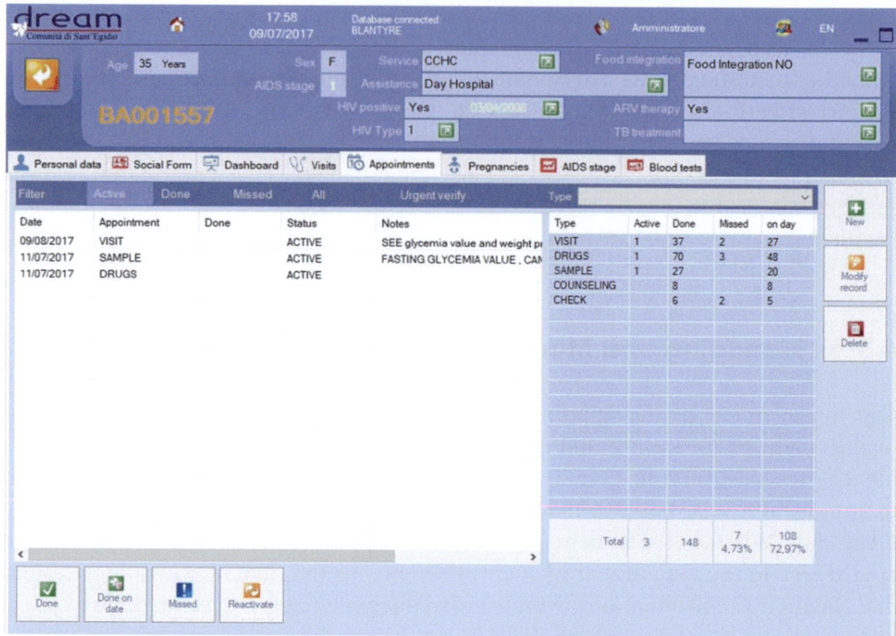

Fig. 4.3 Management of the patients' appointments. Screenshot DREAM® Software (Authorised by ICT DREAM 2017)

antiretroviral drugs, it manages any leftover pills and makes it easier for the pharmacists to dispense appropriate quantities to the patients and to identify the patients who do not adhere adequately (Fig. 4.4).

4.5 Clinical Dashboard

The dashboard has a time graph showing a summary of the patients' clinical history that includes a number of parameters, deriving from clinical observations, laboratory tests, the therapeutic indications and also the medical examinations performed and any pregnancies (Fig. 4.5).

4.6 Monitoring Children's Psychophysical Development

The section regarding the anthropometric and psychophysical development of children is another section in which graphs are very useful. In this section the software uses the data and part of the source code of the WHO Anthro [4] software developed by WHO and made available free of charge to our developers, who integrated it into the DREAM software in order to visualise the anthropometric curves and to point out patients at risk of malnutrition (Fig. 4.6).

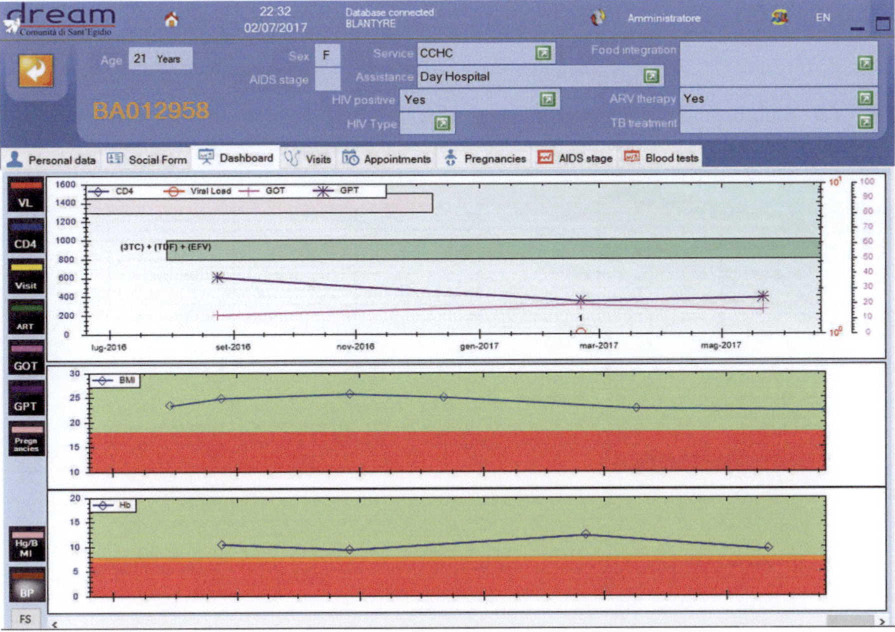

Fig. 4.4 Checking adherence to the antiretroviral therapy for HIV. Screenshot DREAM® Software (Authorised by ICT DREAM 2017)

Fig. 4.5 The dashboard; screenshot DREAM® Software (Authorised by ICT DREAM 2017)

4.7   Clinical Evidence and Management Tools

Another key tool for the overall clinical management of the centre is the "Evidence" section. This section contains several predefined and parametric queries, with which it is possible to test specific samples of patients in the databases. For example, there is a part here that highlights malnutrition issues, and it is possible, for example, to see children with an alarming weight for height ratio or other worrying nutritional indicators (Fig. 4.7).

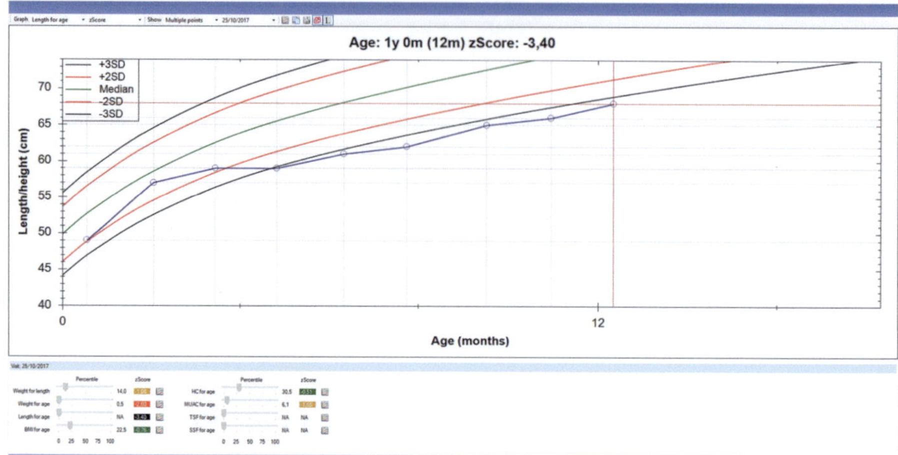

Fig. 4.6 Anthropometric assessment; screenshot DREAM® Software (Authorised by ICT DREAM 2017)

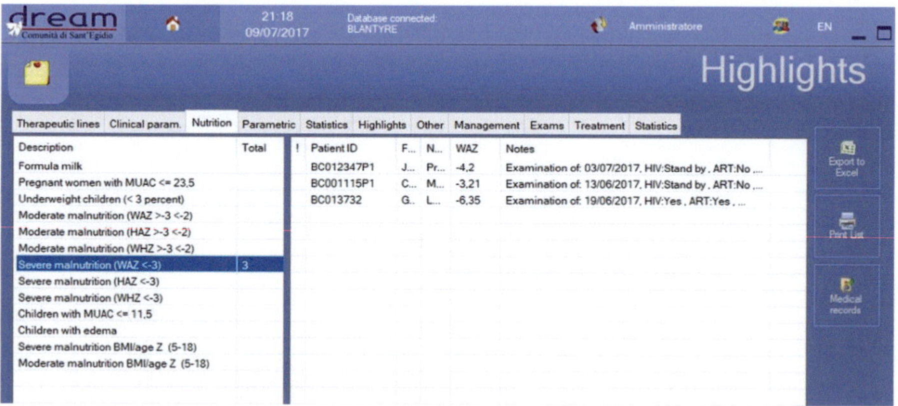

Fig. 4.7 Highlights. Screenshot DREAM® Software (Authorised by ICT DREAM 2017)

With the list produced by this questioning, it is possible to study the anthropometric development of each child in detail, for a better analysis of the alarming value with respect to the children's overall development and in connection to the other information on their medical record. When this assessment has been made, you can go back to the list you started from, to study the next case. This modality is used in particular by the coordinators of the centres in order to identify especially problematic situations or groups of patients to be included in a verification protocol.

It is easy to understand the difference between a simple software that manages the patients' medical records, like EMR, and DREAM software as a point of care. In the first case, it is only possible to assess the patients from a clinical point of

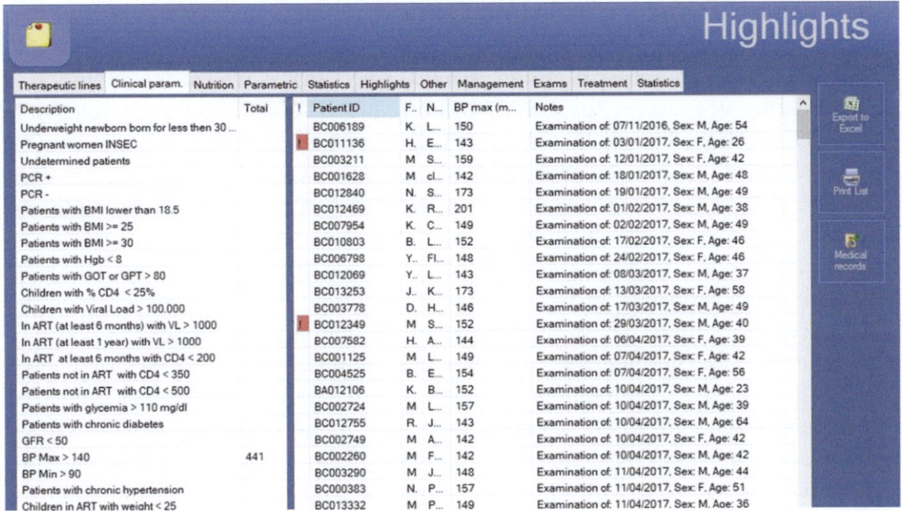

Fig. 4.8 List of patients whose systolic blood pressure is above 140; screenshot DREAM®
Software (Authorised by ICT DREAM 2017)

view, and as far as their adherence is concerned, only when their medical file is
open, one patient at a time. On the other hand, in our case, thanks to the tools
offered by the software, the clinical coordinators and social-healthcare staff can
reach patients with particular problems, in order to highlight specific clinical and
adherence parameters, and they can then draw up lists of people for whom action
needs to be taken.

In the most urgent cases, these patients, who have been identified, are invited to
come to the centre earlier than their next appointment, or else the patients' records
are highlighted with special alerts so that the next time they are accessed, the staff
can see the alert and act accordingly. This function is also essential when you want
to put a specific prevention programme into force. For example, having the possibility to highlight all the patients whose blood pressure is above a certain level can
help define a list of patients to be screened for the prevention of hypertension
(Fig. 4.8).

The software manages several interconnected centres, both from the point of
view of the management of the centres and from that of the patients, who may move
around the country and therefore need to go to a different healthcare centre. Some
functions were therefore implemented, so the patients' electronic medical record
can be transmitted and imported and the requests and reports can be exchanged
between the laboratories and the centres and also the orders and dispensing from the
various storerooms used in the centres regarding the healthcare materials and the
patients' medication.

4.8   The Technological Help Desk

A system like this obviously needs an assistance network as well as the definition of standard setup procedures for the hardware required. Having invested heavily in internet connections has made it possible to act quickly, and when it is not possible to act directly or to solve the problem with computer experts on site, then it is done remotely, with remote, shared, desktop assistance software [5]. For example, the help desk assistance software in Rome provided over 1000 hours of remote assistance in 2016 alone, without counting the thousands of responses provided by the help desk email service.

In conclusion, there has been a reduction of operating times, of the waste of paper and of transcription errors (e.g. by receiving medical records electronically), as a result of the use of computers in every operative unit of the healthcare centres. Consequently the centres work better, and there is more information, which has become easily available, with obvious advantages for both the staff and the patients. The patients are treated with the best equipment, and they also benefit from the systems being computerised because all the procedures are streamlined. Therefore, the patients can go to the centre, for example, with just their identification number and pick up the medication from the pharmacy with their electronic prescription, and they do not have to wait very long because the appointments are organised with the help of the electronic calendar. On the other hand, the staff at the centres are helped from an organisational and a clinical point of view, and they are also gratified by being able to work in an atmosphere that is stimulating from a point of view of innovation, not only medical-scientific but also computer and technological innovation.

References

1. Open-source point-of-care electronic medical records for use in resource-limited settings: systematic review and questionnaire surveys; 2012. https://www.ncbi.nlm.nih.gov/pmc/articles/PMC3391372/
2. A global approach to the management of EMR (Electronic Medical Records) of patients with HIV/AIDS in Sub-Saharan Africa: the experience of DREAM Software. https://www.ncbi.nlm.nih.gov/pmc/articles/PMC2749819/
3. Software open source FlySpray: http://www.flyspray.org
4. http://www.who.int/childgrowth/software/en/
5. Software TeamViewer (http://www.teamviewer.com)

DREAM Centre Remote Telemonitoring   5

Fausto Ciccacci and Giovanni Guidotti

The healthcare model of the DREAM programme necessarily involves the computerisation of its services [1]. Over the years, the computerised management of the programme has been an extremely effective instrument in the centres' everyday work, in order to minimise errors and optimise the quality of the services performed. The DREAM software represents the technological heart of these services. However this computerisation is also useful from many other points of view, and one of these is the centres' remote telemonitoring. The vision behind the DREAM programme is that of a Euro-African response to the enormous challenge of healthcare in Africa, together with a large bet on local staff. In fact there is a great commitment from European professionals in terms of support, training and, in this case, monitoring.

Remote telemonitoring is a long-distance monitoring of the activities of a given health centre that obviously starts with onsite monitoring of the activities. These are two phases, which although they are separate can in practice intersect each other and overlap:

- Onsite monitoring
- Monitoring at a distance (telemonitoring)

Every DREAM centre is managed by several health professionals [2]: doctors, nurses, laboratory technicians, pharmacists, educators and psychologists. The links between the various services are ensured by a coordinator, who is specially trained for this job. The coordinator has to supervise the activities carried out in the various

F. Ciccacci (✉)
'DREAM Program', Community of Sant'Egidio, Rome, Italy
e-mail: fausto.ciccacci@gmail.com

G. Guidotti
Community of Sant'Egidio – DREAM, General Secretary Dream Foundation, Rome, Italy
e-mail: dream@santegidio.org

© Springer International Publishing AG, part of Springer Nature 2018   43
M. Bartolo, F. Ferrari (eds.), *Multidisciplinary Teleconsultation in Developing Countries*, TELe-Health, https://doi.org/10.1007/978-3-319-72763-9_5

sections and make sure that everything is working in harmony. The DREAM software is a very precious instrument for this: every week the coordinator carries out a general check of the centre's activities, using the "evidence" section of the software (see below). This way the first monitoring is carried out onsite, and this is able to direct the work towards the most effective strategies and solve the most obvious and simple management issues.

In theory, all the activities can be monitored at a distance because of the way the DREAM model has been designed, but naturally in practice, only certain issues are analysed periodically [3]. The frequency of these checks and the issues studied can change according to a variety of different factors. Every DREAM centre and every professional who works in a specific site undergo a learning process and continuous training. Consequently the needs vary considerably over time. The activities that have to be monitored when a DREAM centre is first set up are different from those of a centre that has been active for years. In the same way, a centre with only a few patients will have different needs from a centre with thousands of patients, just as a centre that treats many children, or a specialised centre for pregnant women, or a rural centre or one in the city centre, will all have different monitoring needs. Therefore, remote telemonitoring has to have knowledge of the area in which the health centre operates. Generally speaking the people performing the monitoring should know the social context and the availability of other health services in the area and, if possible, also know the staff who work in the centre. While it is true that telemonitoring is monitoring at a distance (and as we will see "at a distance" represents a strong point), it is also true that this distance cannot mean not knowing the context. It is as though it does not make any difference whether the DREAM centre that is monitored is in Maputo, Conakry or Nairobi or even a health centre in Melbourne or Oslo. Although telemonitoring at a distance works along some fixed paths, it cannot be seen as an evaluation grid that is automatically applied to a centre, but rather as a garment that is made to measure for the centre in question, and in order to do this, it is essential to know the measurements of the centre.

The DREAM software is divided into several sections: admission, medical files, blood samples, dispensing drugs, home care, food warehouse, etc.

The section called "highlights" collects the data selected by creating groups according to specific queries (Fig. 5.1).

When checking out this evidence also from remote, a number of different activity parameters may be easily viewed.

The evidence available in the "highlights" section of the software is grouped into topics: nutrition, clinical parameters, therapeutic lines, etc. (Fig. 5.2).

Through these sections, it is possible to identify how many and which patients correspond to specific parameters requested.

The DREAM software developers, together with the doctors and supervisors who are active on the field, identified some indicators that correspond to three main areas:

- The activity statistics of a centre
- Particular case studies to be monitored
- The most frequent clinical and management errors

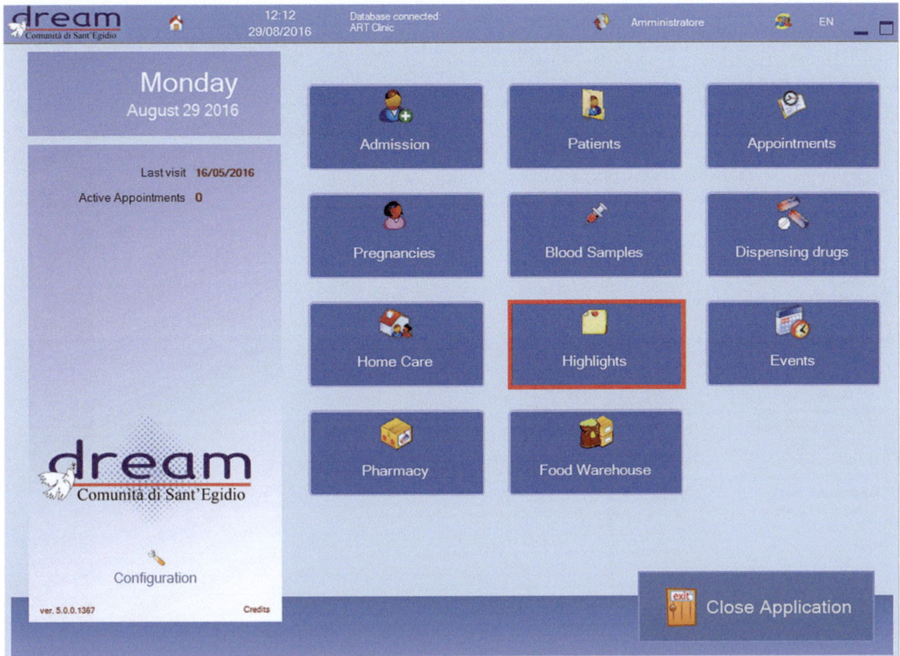

Fig. 5.1 Home page—DREAM software

By now the DREAM programme offers hundreds of indicators and it is not possible to analyse them all. The following example just gives us a general idea of the potential of this software. Some queries, moreover, can be made and saved for the specific requirements of certain clinical centres.

In any case, with this instrument, it is possible to have a rapid overall view of the centre's various activities: the number of patients assisted, how many of them are in the tuberculosis treatment service, the number of women in the mother-to-child HIV prevention programme, the number of HIV tests performed, how many medical examinations have been performed, etc.

It is also possible to identify particular cases that need special follow-up or special attention, for example, patients on a second line of therapy, malnourished children or patients with hypertension, diabetes or kidney or liver failure. These queries will be made by the software so it is possible to carry out specific checks on certain types of patients and highlight any management errors.

The DREAM programme follows specific protocols for every different type of patient. These protocols have been drawn up by infectious disease and public healthcare specialists according to national and international indications. There are specific schedules for medical examinations and blood tests and for handing over the medication.

Every patient has to be assigned to the specific protocol for his/her condition.

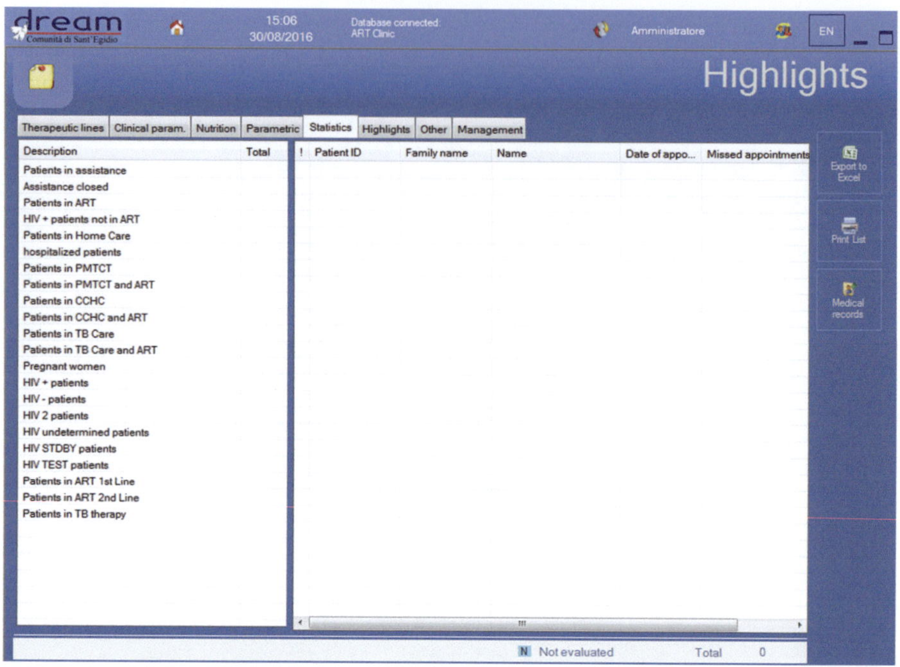

Fig. 5.2 Highlights—DREAM software

For example, patients with TB who receive the antitubercular therapy in the DREAM centre have to have daily or weekly appointments to receive their medication; patients with HIV who are in treatment have to perform the viral load test at least once a year. The "highlights" sections show the cases that do not respect the specific protocols, like patients who do not have any appointments scheduled, patients who receive food integration but are not malnourished, patients whose last viral load test was performed more than 13 months previously, children of women with HIV who do not have a HIV test result at 18 months of age, etc. (Fig. 5.3).

It is clear from these few examples that telemonitoring is one of the strong points of the DREAM programme and it also guarantees constant training and the progress of the healthcare staff who, it is important to remember, are all strictly local.

In the DREAM model, the presence of specialised professionals who monitor the work and who, if necessary, suggest corrections is not perceived as a form of control or a lack of trust in the local staff. The person monitoring is not better than the person who is monitored; they simply do a different job: in fact monitoring requires different professional skills, for example, an overview of the service provided. As often happens, when an outside expert has a look, what they first see are any errors; on the other hand, the people who work locally are involved in their daily routine and are not likely to notice every error.

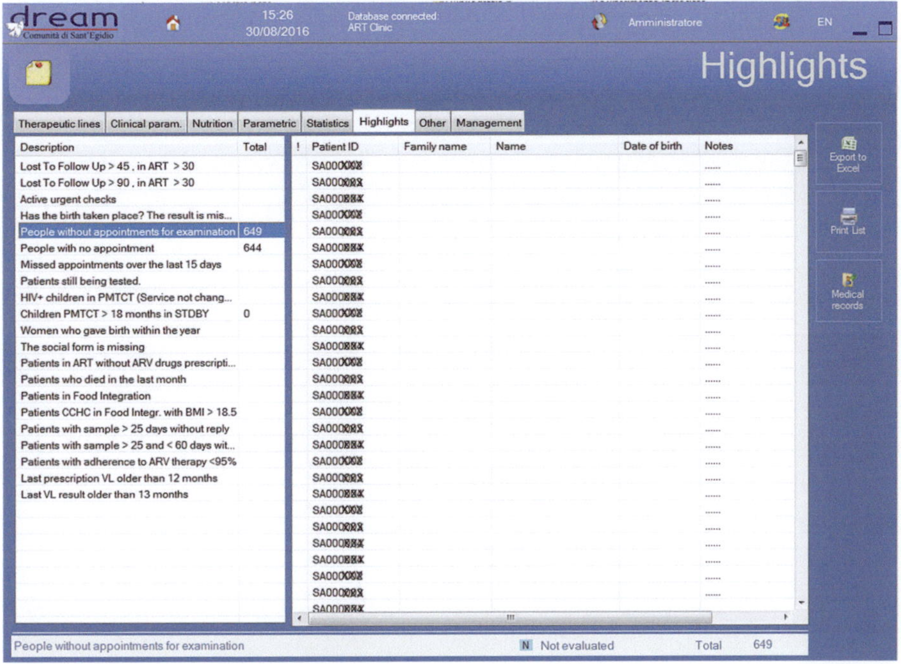

Fig. 5.3 Check some evidence

It is a common experience that when an error that has been made continuously for a long time is pointed out, the answer is "we've always done it that way". Remote telemonitoring makes it possible to quickly identify and correct these issues. Another equally important aspect is that telemonitoring has become a real sort of training at a distance. Correcting, indicating, pointing out issues and explaining any errors are all part of training.

With the growth of the DREAM programme, some local professionals who have been working with the DREAM programme for a long time have also become skilled in telemonitoring. In Mozambique, for example, there are some local professionals who have been regularly performing telemonitoring activities in DREAM centres for years.

References

1. Bartolo M, Nucita A. Telehealth networks for Hospital Services. IGI Global. 2013, p. 97–102.
2. Marazzi C, Buonomo E, Palombi L, et coll. Treating AIDS in Africa. Leonardo International; 2003.
3. AAVV. Long life for Africa: Defeating Aids and malnutrition. Leonardo International; 2008.

DREAM Data Activity

6

Pietro Giglio and Michelangelo Bartolo

DREAM has a 15-year-long history, and in fact the first patients came to the first DREAM centre, in Mozambique in 2002. We immediately realised that we could not provide excellent treatment without recording all the clinical, social and operational data of the healthcare centre quickly, efficiently and systematically. In fact, since the beginning, all this information has been recorded in a database that has grown over the years, and that has made it possible for us to analyse the trend of every healthcare centre. With the data on hand, quickly highlighting the strong points or any critical issues has been a good way to support the medical staff in carefully, accurately and quickly following every patient's clinical history [3, 4].

The data concerning the activities performed is very impressive and expresses the growth of the DREAM programme very well [5, 6].

As the next chapter explains, part of the DREAM programme treats HIV-positive patients. As of June 2017, we have treated over 250,000 patients, 70,000 of whom children, in 11 African countries.

The part of the DREAM programme that deals with the prevention of mother-to-child transmission (PMTCT) has treated just over 100,000 children. Almost ninety-nine percent of them are healthy, and it is thanks to the therapy given to their mothers that they do not have AIDS [7].

Therefore, overall DREAM has treated over 350,000 patients since 2002.

These figures have been achieved with a slow but constant increase in the number of patients treated, which can be seen in detail in the table and in the graph below (Table 6.1 and Fig. 6.1).

P. Giglio (✉)
'DREAM Program', Community of Sant'Egidio, Rome, Italy
e-mail: piero.giglio@gmail.com

M. Bartolo
Telemedicine Unit, San Giovanni Hospital, Rome, Italy
e-mail: michelebartolo@gmail.com

© Springer International Publishing AG, part of Springer Nature 2018

49

M. Bartolo, F. Ferrari (eds.), *Multidisciplinary Teleconsultation in Developing Countries*, TELe-Health, https://doi.org/10.1007/978-3-319-72763-9_6

Table 6.1 Number of patients treated; data provided by ICT DREAM 2017

Year	M	F	Total
2003–2004	3115	5787	8902
2005	6514	11,914	18,428
2006	8981	17,175	26,156
2007	15,804	31,534	47,338
2008	22,481	49,641	72,122
2009	34,221	70,553	104,774
2010	41,328	87,949	129,277
2011	45,149	95,315	140,464
2012	51,591	107,264	158,855
2013	60,427	126,323	186,750
2014	66,658	142,583	209,241
2015	71,160	151,697	222,857
2016	75,639	161,897	237,536
2017	81,131	169,721	250,852

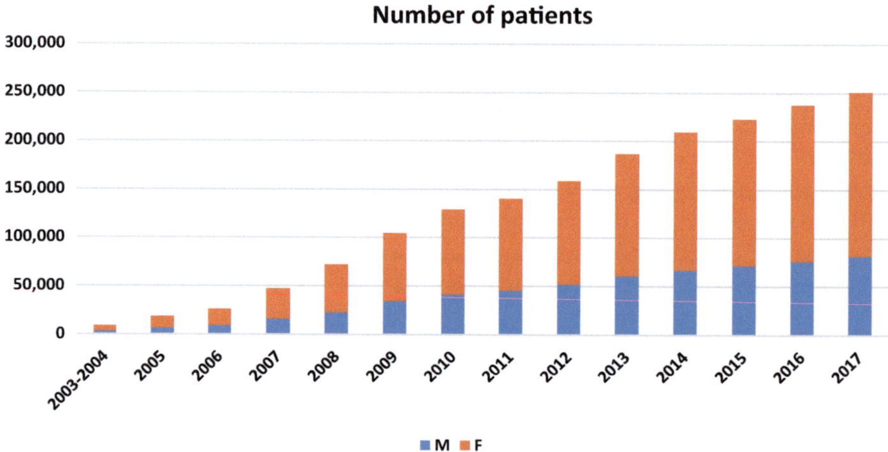

Fig. 6.1 Number of patients treated; data provided by ICT DREAM 2017

Looking at these figures, one fact stands out immediately; there are twice as many women as men. This fact obviously does not reflect the epidemiology of the disease, but it indicates that women are generally more inclined to receive the treatment than men. Women are responsible for their families and their children, so the fact that there are more women in our healthcare centres is a clear example of this characteristic of African women, who accept to take the therapy in order to guarantee a future for their children.

The number of activities shows the vast amount of work that has been carried out over the years by the medical staff, the nurses, laboratory technicians and the coordinators who, it is important to remember, are all local staff. However it is also important to remember that this effort to grow would not be possible without a large number of European volunteers, who have performed most of the work

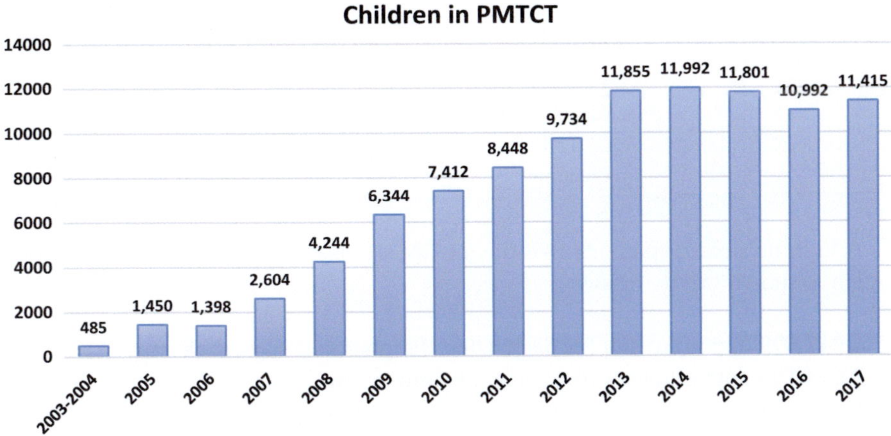

Fig. 6.2 DREAM data: children born in PMTCT. Data provided by ICT DREAM 2017

Table 6.2 DREAM data: children born in PMTCT. Data provided by ICT DREAM 2017

Years	Children in *PMTCT*
2003–2004	485
2005	1450
2006	1398
2007	2604
2008	4244
2009	6344
2010	7412
2011	8448
2012	9734
2013	11,855
2014	11,992
2015	11,801
2016	10,992
2017	11,415
Total	100,174

described in this book. A detailed analysis of the PMTCT programme also shows a constant growth of this part of the programme (Fig. 6.2 and Table 6.2).

The number of children born in the vertical prevention programme (PMTCT) immediately shows how effective the programme is. From 2002 to today, 100,174 children were born, of whom almost 99% tested HIV negative. The data reveal how it is possible to protect a whole generation from the transmission of HIV. Over 100,000 children represent a new generation that are a witness to the fact that HIV can be fought and defeated by prevention.

Table 6.3 DREAM activity lab data. Data provided by ICT DREAM 2017

Tests from the beginning of DREAM	
CD4	942,263
Viral load	793,706
Haemoglobin	1,309,652
GOT/GPT	1,018,586
Creatinine	709,964

A high number of patients like this obviously involve a great amount of work, which is shown briefly below:

- **4,047,899** appointments for dispensing the pharmacological therapy
- **2,614,100** appointments for medical examinations
- **1,637,305** appointments for taking blood samples

The data below show the extent of the vast amount of work that has also been performed by the molecular biology laboratories for the healthcare centres. The graph shows that almost 950,000 CD4 tests have been carried out and almost 800,000 viral load measurements, 1,300,000 haemoglobin tests and over one million GOT and GPT tests have been performed (Table 6.3).

Today the DREAM programme is present in 11 sub-Saharan African countries: Mozambique, Swaziland, Malawi, Tanzania, Kenya, Central African Republic, Democratic Republic of Congo, Guinea Conakry, Cameroon, Nigeria and Angola.

References

1. Emberti Gialloreti L, Palombi L, Buonomo E, Guidotti G, Nathave I, Liotta G, Marazzi MC. Pilot programme for prevention and treatment of AIDS in Mozambique. XII International Conference on AIDS and STDs in Africa, 9–13/12/2001, Ouagadougou, Burkina Faso. Abs Book, p 59, N.10 pt 3–206
2. Liotta G, Mancinelli S, Riccardi F, Palombi L, Marazzi MC, Narciso P, Emberti Gialloreti L. A protocol for the therapy of HIV infection and the prevention of mother-to-child transmission in Mozambique. XIV International AIDS Conference, Barcellona 7–12–Jul 2002. Vol II, D11394.
3. Andrea Nucita, Giuseppe M Bernava, Michelangelo Bartolo, Fabio Di Pane Masi, Pietro Giglio, Marco Peroni, Giovanni Pizzimenti and Leonardo Palombi. Global approach to the management of EMR (Electronic Medical Records) of patients with HIV/AIDS in Sub-Saharan Africa: the experience of DREAM Software.
4. Benefits and challenges of EMR implementations in low resource settings: a state-of-the-art review https://www.ncbi.nlm.nih.gov/pmc/articles/PMC5011989/
5. Telemedicine for HIV Prevention and Treatment in Sub-Saharan Africa – M. Bartolo – Community of Sant'Egidio, Telemedicine Manager S. Giovanni, M. Peroni, S. Benedetti. P. Del Bove, A. Nucita, F. Di Pane, G.M. Bernava – Community of Sant'Egidio, L. Palombi – University of Tor Vergata – Rome, P. Giglio – DREAM Program.
6. Marazzi MC, Palombi L, Gennaro E, Buonomo E, Scarcella P, Mancinelli S, Doro Altan AM, Ceffa S, Staniscia T, Lotta G. Epidemia da HIV/AIDS: il potenziale ruolo protettivo della HAART (Highly Active Antiretroviral Therapy) nel controllo della mortalità materna. Risultati del Programma DREAM. Atti della XII Conferenza Nazionale di Sanità Pubblica. Roma 12–15 ottobre 2011. Comunicazione 583, p. 429.

7. Liotta G, Marazzi M, Mothibi K, Zimba I, Amangoua E, Bonje E, Bossiky B, Robinson P, Scarcella P, Musokotwane K, Palombi L, Germano P, Narciso P, de Luca A, Alumando E, Mamary S, Magid N, Guidotti G, Mancinelli S, Orlando S, Peroni M, Buonomo E, Nielsen-Saines K. Elimination of mother-to-child transmission of HIV infection: the drug resource enhancement against AIDS and malnutrition model. Int J Environ Res Public Health. 2015;12 (12):13224–13239.

DREAM 2.0 A Replicable Model

7

Paola Germano and Abdul Majid Noorjehan

7.1 DREAM Replicable

As we fully explained in Chap. 3, when we started working on the DREAM programme, many people considered our dream to take the AIDS therapy to Africa, a utopia: a beautiful, ambitious project but impossible to carry out. Over the years the interest shown throughout the world and the funds raised to fight the disease have not only led to the development of new groups of drugs but also to a greater possibility of diagnosis and treatment in many areas of the world, including Africa.

Today, over a decade later, also thanks to DREAM, which has the merit of having created a model that can be adapted and replicated, by now it is possible to prevent and treat HIV/AIDS in every country in Africa.

The rapid expansion of DREAM over the last 16 years is due not only to the widespread presence of the Community of Sant'Egidio in many countries in Africa and to the work of many African health professionals but also to the collaboration with many religious congregations, NGOs and volunteers who decided to join us in the fight against AIDS. This synergy made it possible to increase the number of patients we can reach. In order to convince many sceptical sick people to accept treatment, we also cooperated with the communities of other religions and denominations, for example, the Muslim community in Guinea Conakry, with the Hindu community in Malawi or with the Protestant and Orthodox churches in Mozambique. One can say there was a positive effect, which multiplied the effectiveness of our work. This positive effect derives from high-quality healthcare,

P. Germano (✉)
'DREAM Program', Community of Sant'Egidio, Rome, Italy
e-mail: paolagermano1@gmail.com

A. M. Noorjehan
'DREAM Program', Community of Sant'Egidio, Maputo, Mozambique
e-mail: nurjamajid@yahoo.com

© Springer International Publishing AG, part of Springer Nature 2018
M. Bartolo, F. Ferrari (eds.), *Multidisciplinary Teleconsultation in Developing Countries*, TELe-Health, https://doi.org/10.1007/978-3-319-72763-9_7

which has not only made Africa better but also people from many other wealthy parts of the world.

However DREAM is not only the result of projects designed by expert clinical doctors and scientific researchers, but it is also the result of collaboration between people in the north and in the south of the world, including specialists and patients, lay and religious people, volunteers and professionals and donors and governments. This has created a single vision that provides greater strength, and everyone has their own role in order to deal with this terrible pandemic (from home-care assistants to biologists, doctors, logistic staff, nurses and the patients who support other patients who are on the treatment programme). Our ability to discuss difficulties with local people and find solutions to any sort of problem that comes up along the way makes it possible to avoid starting all over again in every country, and in fact it is possible to grow together quickly, by learning from the experiences of other health centres. This permanent relationship, which is not only professional but also friendly, between people in the north and people in the south of the world makes it possible to optimise the system quickly and offer high standards, even when a new centre is set up and the staff is almost completely new.

This also explains the exponential growth of DREAM and the increase in the number of health centres in 11 countries of sub-Saharan Africa (graph). The centres can be replicated, with a few differences, but they all have some essential features that are an inherent part of DREAM.

7.1.1 Excellence

Excellence is one of the concepts that guides DREAM:

1. Excellence in diagnostics, for example, in the introduction of the measurement of the viral load for HIV patients or the more general use of highly specialised molecular biology laboratories
2. Excellence in staff training, the use of the latest generation therapies, no longer substandard or a minimum amount
3. Excellence in terms of the ICT, the installations, the stable electricity supply also from solar panels and better solutions for ensuring an internet connection even in the most remote areas of Africa

These latter aspects are dealt with in other chapters.

7.1.2 The Centrality of the Patient

Continuous research for efficacy in managing the patients is carried out because it is the patient who is the priority. The starting point is men and women and not the institutions. The patient is taken into consideration as a whole, with a holistic approach [1]. Africans with AIDS are complex cases and are not a photocopy of the people with AIDS who live in rich countries; one has to get to know them, listen to them and study them and also respond to their needs in terms of prevention, therapy and also to their social needs. They often have opportunistic infections, they always have to be assessed from a nutritional point of view, and when they need it, they are offered food integration as therapy so that they can have enough to eat for their treatment to be effective. African patients often need health education, they have to be motivated to adhere to the treatment programme, and often they have to be helped to be accepted by their family and their social environment again. By listening to the patients and through continuous contact with them, the patients have been central figures in DREAM's growth and its adherence to the African reality. DREAM in fact represents one of Africa's positive aspects, not only with respect to its approach to health and science but even more from the human point of view, which is what really characterises it.

7.1.3 A Caring Community

DREAM has enhanced and organised a typically African attitude by creating a caring community around the patients with a strongly inclusive approach. In its vision and in practice, the health centre is the place where people come out of isolation and meet other people. It is a place where they are welcomed, where they are listened to and where they have the chance to talk about and express their desire to be cured. Basically it is a place, as well as being a medical health centre, where the patients are encouraged to socialise and become part of society again.

The social work carried out in the centres is resolute and unceasing.

There are an incredible number of meetings with the patients and not only for purely health reasons or related to the diagnostic and therapeutic protocols. The patients are contacted for a variety of reasons including counselling, to take part in meetings and health education, to receive food and medication and then naturally for medical examinations and laboratory tests. All these activities, some of which are typically African, are managed, suggested and planned by the DREAM software, which we could call "software with a human face".

7.1.4 Health Is Not Only Healthcare

For DREAM, the WHO definition that health is not only the absence of pathology is absolutely true [2]. Many factors that have nothing to do with healthcare contribute to determine the state of health of populations: level of education, income, access to food and water, the dramatic consequences of increases in food prices and periods of draught all affect people's state of health.

What is equally important is each patient's context in terms of personal relationships. Coming out of isolation is the first step in the healing process. The aim of eliminating the stigma, which excludes patients from any social life, by creating community networks, is not only an ethical but also a health priority.

A patient who is isolated, demotivated, alone and an outcast often stops adhering to the treatment, and administering the treatment intermittently is pointless and can be even dangerous.

"Taking care" of others is one of the values of the programme.

7.1.5 The Patients as Central Figures

In DREAM the patients are not only the people who use a healthcare service, but they also play an active role as central figures in the DREAM programme. Many of them, in particular the women, decide to actively help other sick people. They become real witnesses, and they carry out irreplaceable work providing support, counselling and peer education and fighting the stigma [3]. They tell people that AIDS is not a death sentence, and they work personally in advertising campaigns against the stigma. The commitment and testimonies of many of these women have brought thousands of people to the therapy. Some of them even have access to part of the DREAM software so they can organise and monitor the home-care service. Moreover, all the patients in the programme attend health education courses, which foster an awareness of community health by teaching people how to deal with many different aspects of life properly, for example, nutrition, use of drinking water, personal hygiene, house cleaning and child care. With this wealth of knowledge, the patients in turn become educators for their families and for the people around them; it gives them a deeper understanding of the causes and mechanisms of diseases, which frees them of fear. The patients become central figures in their own treatment and in other people's treatment. This aspect of the programme is also the key to success in fighting other diseases in Africa. In this fight to save human lives, reduce the spread of many infectious diseases and reduce mortality, education is a very powerful weapon and an extraordinary instrument, which greatly improves our capacity to deal with various pathologies.

The activities briefly explained above are described in a book [4] that has been translated into several languages. This is the story of Pacem Kawonga, a Malawian woman who talks about how she was brought back to life and has since then worked hard so that other people can have the therapy too [5].

7.1.6 The Fight Against Malnutrition

DREAM also actively fights hunger and malnutrition. One section of the software follows the children's psychophysical development; it automatically calculates the growth curves and shows the parameters that are necessary for monitoring the children's growth in order to interrupt the vicious cycle of malnutrition and HIV/AIDS.

Nutritional support is considered just as important as the pharmacological therapy. With the software it is possible to manage the food storeroom and hand out the food packages to specific patients, and the food can also be adapted to different countries [6].

7.1.7 Light Healthcare

DREAM uses light healthcare. Rather than build large hospitals, there is widespread network of excellent health clinics and reference centres for patients from day hospitals located in the most remote and rural areas. Intermediate level services are offered here, like checking and distributing medication and carrying out some types of tests. There are also mobile clinics and home care, which makes access to therapy possible for everyone, even in the most remote villages.

7.1.8 Free of Charge

Everyone can access the DREAM programme because the diagnostics, the therapy and the assistance are all completely free of charge. Africa is a continent with hundreds of millions of people living in extreme poverty, so we had no choice. As well as the fact that hardly anyone has any money, there is also the fact that the therapy lasts a lifetime and the patients have to adhere to it. In any case, the complexity of the assistance, which consists in a high number of appointments for checking on the patients' health, handing over medication and carrying out tests, is costly for the patients. In fact many of them have to travel long distances to get to the centres for all their appointments, and this takes a long time. This has a cost: nobody receives contributions for transport, and in fact adhering to the treatment involves the active participation of the patients, who participate indirectly from an economic point of view.

The DREAM programme has to be free of charge first of all because it is a question of equality and fairness, but it is also the secret of the patients' extremely high degree of adherence to the therapy, which today is considered what really makes the difference in the success of the therapy.

Offering the treatment free of charge is the first way to break down that wall that separates the rich people who can afford healthcare services and the poor.

In these times of globalisation, faced with the challenge of living together and crushed by materialism, the concept of offering services free of charge represents a revolutionary gesture that encourages social development; it gives a boost to the culture of solidarity, voluntary work and cooperation; and it generates new dimensions for our society, without which humanity becomes barbaric. Living in changing times and being able to face the current challenges of a complex and globalised world also means preserving and promoting our humanitarian side. There is something that cannot be sold and cannot be bought, but it is crucial for our lives. This is love, friendship, giving and offering free of charge, which constitute the quality of society and of people's lives. This builds concrete solidarity between people, and it changes the world.

These are the keys to success that explain the rapid spread of DREAM and the reason why it can be replicated.

References

1. Comunità di Sant'Egidio. Dream. Curare l'Aids in Africa. Leonardo International; 2009.
2. Secondo la costituzione dell'OMS la salute è "uno stato di completo benessere fisico, mentale e sociale e non la semplice assenza dello stato di malattia o infermità". Constitution of the World Health Organization, adottata alla International Health Conference tenutasi a New York tra il 19 giugno e il 22 luglio 1946, e firmata il 22 luglio 1946 dai rappresentanti di 61 stati.
3. Programma DREAM, Comunità di Sant'Egidio, Viva l'Africa viva! Vicnere l'AIDS e la malnutrizione Leonardo International; 2008.
4. Comunità di Sant'Egidio Como vai a saúde Leonardo International; 2004.
5. Kawonga P. Un domani per i mei bambini Piemme; 2013.
6. World Food Programme. DREAM programme DREAM: an integrated public health programme to fight HIV/AIDS and malnutrition in limited-resource settings; Ottobre 2007.

The Challenge of Sustainability: The Impact of DREAM Programme on the Social, Economic and Working Conditions of Patients with HIV/AIDS

8

Stefano Orlando

Abbreviations

AIDS	Acquired immunodeficiency syndrome
ARV	Antiretroviral
BMI	Body mass index
CSDH	Commission on Social Determinants of Health
VL	Viral load
DALY	Disability-adjusted life years
DREAM	Drug Resource Enhancement against AIDS and Malnutrition
HAART	Highly active antiretroviral treatment
Hb	Haemoglobin
HDI	Human Development Index
HIV	Human immunodeficiency virus
LPS	Livestock price survey
MWK	Malawian Kwacha
NAC	National Aids Commission (Malawi)
NACP	National AIDS Control Programme (Malawi)
GDP	Gross domestic product
LDC	Least developed countries
PPP	Purchasing power parity
UN	United Nations
UNAIDS	Joint United Nations Programme on HIV/AIDS
UNDP	United Nations Development Programme
UNFPA	United Nations Population Fund

S. Orlando (✉)
University Tor Vergata, Rome, Italy
e-mail: stefano.orlando@uniroma2.it

© Springer International Publishing AG, part of Springer Nature 2018
M. Bartolo, F. Ferrari (eds.), *Multidisciplinary Teleconsultation in Developing Countries*, TELe-Health, https://doi.org/10.1007/978-3-319-72763-9_8

UNICEF   United Nations Children's Fund
WB   World Bank
WHO   World Health Organization

8.1   Introduction

Over the last three decades, the health systems of less developed countries (LDC), which were already very weak and unable to satisfy their citizens' basic needs, have been put to the test because of the HIV/AIDS pandemic, which has hit the countries of sub-Saharan Africa in particular.

HIV/AIDS represents a serious social problem. The pandemic has a strong impact on the societies and on the economies of the countries that are most badly affected by the virus [1]. In the LDCs the pandemic is gradually thwarting the progress towards development which, despite countless difficulties, was slowly happening over the last years.

The negative impact of the AIDS pandemic on economic growth has been widely studied [2–4]. However the question remains: what is the best approach for reduction of the effects of the pandemic and possible elimination of the virus?

The evaluation of the cost-effectiveness or cost-benefit ratios is therefore a fundamental aspect in evaluating the best approach to adopt in fighting AIDS and especially how to assess the sustainability of HIV/AIDS programmes. In the literature however, there are only a few evaluations of the positive impact of AIDS treatment programmes adopted to reduce its negative effect on health [5–7] and on the economy [8–10].

This chapter analyses the impact of the DREAM programme that mixes antiretroviral therapy with a range of correlated services (psychosocial support, health education, nutritional support), on the social, economic and working conditions of HIV+ patients.

ARV (antiretroviral) therapy, administered correctly, greatly reduces morbidity and mortality in people with HIV, both in developed countries [11–14] and in LDC [15–18].

The treatment has a positive impact on income first of all because it makes it possible for people who had been weakened by the disease to be reintegrated into the workforce, thus increasing the work offer, and secondly because together with increased income, there is also a reduction in expenses related to the disease; therefore both public and private savings and investments increase, both in terms of physical capital and human capital. So it is advisable, also in order to provide a useful instrument for cost-benefit analyses in this field, to analyse the impact of the programme on the work offer and average income.

In this analysis, the study population was selected from a cohort of patients enrolled in the DREAM programme in Malawi, in two ART centres both in rural and urban settings (the Mtemgowamtemga centre in the rural area of Dowa, Lilongwe and the Blantyre centre, the largest trading town, respectively) with the following inclusion criteria: HIV positivity, age >15 and ART initiation within 2 months of enrolment.

Forms provided by the Medical Outcomes Study HIV Health Survey (MOS-HIV) [19] and WHO performance questionnaires [20] were used to design the questionnaire. General principles used in social research questionnaires were also applied [21]. These forms were then adapted to meet specific requirements for this study. The income was reported by respondents in Malawi Kwacha and then converted to USD at purchasing power parity (PPP) using criteria adopted by the WHO for economic analysis in health programmes [22]. A patient self-evaluation of their own health and economic status was taken into consideration to counterpose information coming from the economic data.

Most of the people selected were women (70%). Nonetheless this composition of the study population reflects the general situation regarding HAART recipients in sub-Saharan Africa [23].

A total number of 165 subjects were followed from January 2008 to March 2009. All subjects had at least 8 months of follow-up post-ART initiation.

A certain loss was observed at the follow-up (23%), mainly due to the patients' work and social mobility. Nonetheless, considering the low number of people lost to follow-up, and considering the fact that the cause of this loss did not concern their state of health, these patients were excluded from the analysis. The patients who were excluded presented a similar state of health and economic situation as those who were included.

Health, income and productivity parameters were evaluated through paired t-test.

8.2   Results

The overall health status of subjects improved significantly based on clinical and virologic parameters (see Table 8.1).

The main impact observed was in the variation of mean HIV-1 RNA (viral load). In fact this parameter reacted to therapy before the other ones, which has biological plausibility. Nonetheless there was also a significant difference in mean CD4 cell count levels. Since this parameter measures the strength of the person's immune system, it is a clear indicator of his/her state of health. In fact it is more likely that a person with a high viral load (negative information) but who also has a high number of CD4 cells will feel better than a person with a low number of CD4 cells and a low viral load. Actually, the most predictive variable of good health is the BMI (body mass index). Nonetheless this variable responds more slowly to therapy, and above all it is greatly influenced by external factors like a good diet. Although the haemoglobin value is strongly related to antiretroviral treatment, it can also be influenced by many other factors.

Looking at the socio-economic data generated, a positive overall impact on productivity and income was noted. Hours worked in the last week increased by 25%, hours worked in the last month increased by 31%, income generated in the last week increased by 85%, and income in the last month increased by 80% (Table 8.2).

Table 8.1 Clinical and virologic parameters of the sample

| Variables | Mean value Baseline (t0) | Mean value Follow-up (t1) | Mean increase and % change | 95% confidence interval of difference | | |
				Min	Max	P
Malnutrition (BMI)	21.38	21.79	0.10 (12%)	0.03	0.18	0.009
Haemoglobin	11.61	12.99	0.20 (11%)	0.10	0.29	<0.001
CD4 cell count (cells/mm^3)	276	379	0.47 (62%)	0.35	0.59	<0.001
HIV-1 RNA Log10	3.93	0.71	1.37 (285%)	1.20	1.53	<0.001

Table 8.2 Impact of treatment on work offer and income

| Variables | Mean value Baseline (t0) | Mean value Follow-up (t1) | Mean increase and % change | 95% confidence interval of difference | | |
				Min	Max	P
Hours worked last 7 days	24	30	6 (25%)	1	11	<0.05
Hours worked last 30 days	96	126	30 (31%)	13	48	<0.01
Income over last 7 days	10.93	20.25	9.31 (85%)	1.45	17.17	<0.05
Income over last 30 days	43.97	79.29	35.32 (80%)	11.88	58.76	<0.01

For patients who were unemployed at baseline (n = 37), mean income was too low (<4\$ per month) to be relevant for the analysis. With the exclusion of unemployed patients at baseline, the increase in last week/last month hours worked was +35% and +43%, respectively, and last week/last month income +93% and +89%, respectively (+400\$ per year).

8.2.1 Patient Self-Evaluation

The patient's answers to control questions asked during the second round of interviews confirmed the results of the analysis. The answers regarding their economic condition are distributed along a normal curve (Fig. 8.1); however, looking at answers regarding the variation of their economic situation with respect to the previous 10 months (Fig. 8.2), most patients interviewed said their situation had improved (43.3%), and only 25.3% said that it was worse. One has to bear in

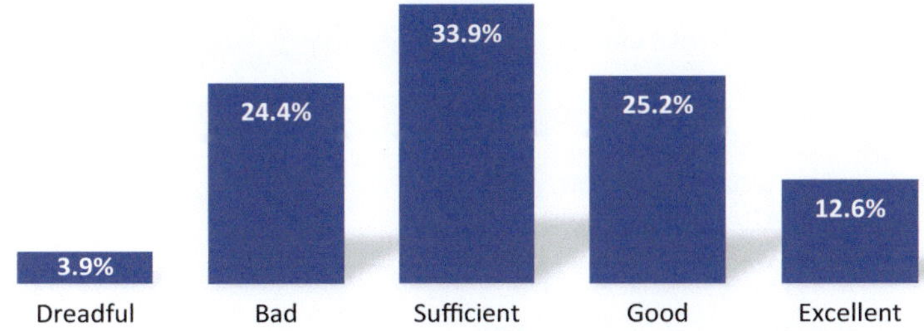

Fig. 8.1 Perceived economic situation

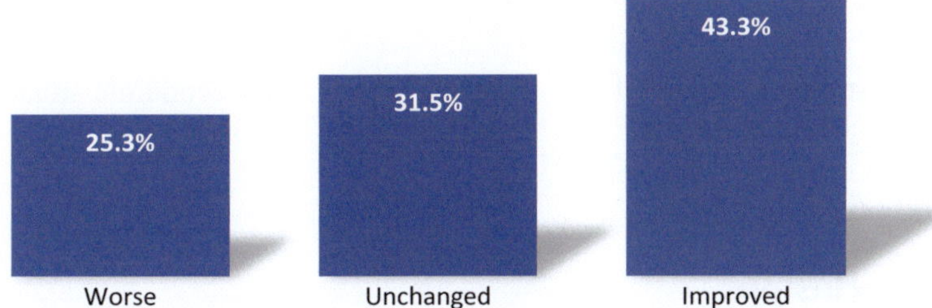

Fig. 8.2 Perception of variation in economic situation

mind that these were ill people and that over the period during which the interviews were carried out, there was a serious economic crisis that hit many African countries and in particular the most vulnerable populations. In fact the crisis was caused by an increase in the cost of fuel, and therefore of transport, and by the rapid and high increase in the price of cereals, the basic element of the Malawian diet. This crisis set off revolutions in Malawi and also in neighbouring countries. So it is remarkable that in such a serious situation, and on a sample of people who are vulnerable because of disease, less than one third of the subjects said that their situation had become worse.

Once the socio-economic situation of the study population was assessed through the variation in work offer and income, there was still the problem of characterising health, that is, improvement in health due to AIDS treatment, as the main cause of this phenomenon. It was considered appropriate to evaluate whether the patients themselves considered their state of health an important reason, if not the main reason, for the changes in their socio-economic situation. Those who said there had not been any particular changes in their situation over the previous 8 months were excluded from the analysis.

The answers reported in Fig. 8.3 indicated health as the main reason behind both positive and negative changes (54.6%); 46.5% said their health improved and also their economic situation. However 7% said that their health improved but that their economic situation did not. This reflects what was mentioned before that, during the study period, there was an economic crisis in Malawi, so even though the health of

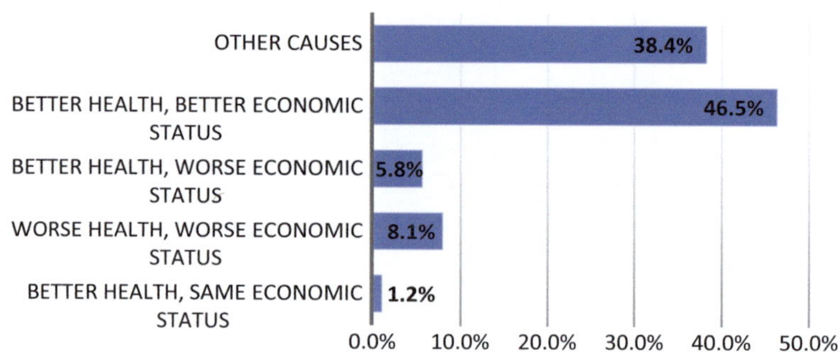

Fig. 8.3 Causes of variation in economic situation

participating subjects improved, due to other reasons, their economic situation did not improve.

8.3   Conclusions

The main objective of this study was to measure the impact of HIV/AIDS treatment administered in the DREAM programme on one of the most important aspects of development and economic growth: productivity, that is, work offer and increase in income. Of course income is just one of the factors involved in economic development, and the HIV/AIDS epidemic also reduces development through its impact on other fundamental factors. Nonetheless this is one of the aspects of development where the outcomes of actions taken to counter the disease can be noted and measured.

The mean increase of approximately USD400 is very important within a cost/benefit analysis. The cost of antiretroviral therapy, including the diagnostics, in large-scale programmes using generic drugs, is in fact around this value per year. This means that the cost of therapy is completely covered simply because of the increase in income due to therapy itself. However this calculation does not take into consideration the fact that without therapy the patient's health would probably get worse, so his capacity to work would be further reduced. The decline in productivity due to the worsening of the state of health cannot be measured directly because ethical issues would arise. In fact, a control group should be monitored, which would not be given therapy even if needed. The value of this loss should be added to the benefit derived from the therapy estimated at USD600. This study does not even calculate the indirect effects of this action, for example, related to the savings for the state in terms of hospitalisation costs for the patients, the costs saved by the companies with respect to the turnover of employees due to high mortality, the impact on public expenditures and income tax and all the other negative effects of AIDS described in Chap. 1.

In conclusion, the treatment of AIDS is completely sustainable from an economic point of view; actually it can really be considered an investment with a high return in human capital.

References

1. Piot P, Bartos M, Ghys P, et al. The global impact of HIV/AIDS. Nature. 2001;410:968–73.
2. Haacker M. Modeling the macroeconomic impact of HIV/AIDS. IMF Working Papers (International Monetary Fund), 195; 2002.
3. Haacker M. The economic consequences of HIV/AIDS in Southern Africa. IMF Working Papers (International Monetary Fund), 38; 2002.
4. Bell C, Devarajan S, Gersbach H et al. The long-run economic costs of AIDS: theory and an application to South Africa. The World Bank; 2003.
5. Coetzee D, Hildebrand K, Boulle A, et al. Outcomes after two years of providing antiretroviral treatment in Khayelitsha, South Africa. AIDS. 2004;18(6):887–95.
6. Ferradini L, et al. Scaling up of highly active antiretroviral therapy in a rural district of Malawi: an effectiveness assessment. The Lancet. 2006;367(9519):1335–42.
7. Bekker L, Myer L, Orrell C, Lawn S, et al. Rapid scale-up of a community-based HIV treatment service. S Afr Med J. 2006;96(4):315–22.
8. Larson B, Fox M, Rosen S, et al. Early effects of antiretroviral therapy on work performance: preliminary results from a cohort study of Kenyan agricultural workers. AIDS. 2008;22 (3):421–5.
9. Rosen S, Ketlhapile M, Sanne I, et al. Differences in normal activities, job performance and symptom prevalence between patients not yet on antiretroviral therapy and patients initiating therapy in South Africa. AIDS. 2008;22(Suppl 1):S131–9.
10. Thirumurthy H, Zivin JG, Goldstein M. The economic impact of AIDS treatment: labor supply in Western Kenya. J Hum Resour. 2008;43(3):511–52.
11. Palella F, Delaney K, Moorman A. Declining morbidity and mortality among patients with advanced human immunodeficiency virus infection. N Engl J Med. 1998;338(13):853–60.
12. Hogg R, Heath K, Yip B. Improved survival among HIV-infected individuals following initiation of antiretroviral therapy. JAMA. 1998;279(6):450–4.
13. Hammer S, Squires K, Hughes M. A controlled trial of two nucleoside analogues plus indinavir in persons with human immunodeficiency virus infection and CD4 cell counts of 200 per cubic millimeter or less. N Engl J Med. 1997;337(11):725–33.
14. Hunt P, Deeks S, Rodriguez B, et al. Continued CD4 cell count increases in HIV-infected adults experiencing 4 years of viral suppression on antiretroviral therapy. AIDS. 2003;17 (13):1907–15.
15. Laurent C, Diakhaté N, Gueye NF, et al. The Senegalese government's highly active antiretroviral therapy initiative: an 18-month follow-up study. AIDS. 2002;16(10):1363–70.
16. Marins J, Jamal L, Chen S, et al. Dramatic improvement in survival among adult Brazilian AIDS patients. AIDS. 2003;17(11):1675–82.
17. Koenig S, Leandre F, Farmer P. Scaling-up HIV treatment programmes in resource-limited settings: the rural Haiti experience. AIDS. 2004;18:S21–5.
18. Wools-Kaloustian K, Kimaiyo S, Diero L, et al. Viability and effectiveness of large-scale HIV treatment initiatives in sub-Saharan Africa: experience from western Kenya. AIDS. 2006;20 (1):41–8.
19. Wu AW, Revicki DA, Jacobson D, et al. Evidence for reliability, validity and usefulness of the Medical Outcomes Study HIV Health Survey (MOS-HIV). Qual Life Res (Springer). 1997;6:481–93.
20. Kessler RC. World Health Organization Health and Performance Questionnaire (HPQ): clinical trials baseline version. Geneva: World Health Organization; 2002.
21. De Vaus D. Surveys in social research. Oxon: Routledge; 2002.
22. http://www.who.int/choice/costs/ppp/en/
23. Pienaar D, Myer L, Cleary S. Models of care for antiretroviral service delivery. Cape Town, South Africa: University of Cape Town; 2006.

Part III

GHT, Remote Healthcare

Multispecialist Teleconsultation

Michelangelo Bartolo and Fabio Ferrari

When Global Health Telemedicine started in 2008, with the first telemedicine centre in Arusha, in Tanzania [1], nobody would have expected that in just a few years, there would be such a great increase in demand, for teleconsultations and also to open new centres. Today GHT is present in 12 African countries, with 29 telemedicine centres (Fig. 9.1).

Most of these telemedicine stations were set up in the Community of Sant'Egidio's DREAM healthcare centres. In fact GHT was created as a result of the DREAM programme with the aim to provide a platform for rapid communication between the doctors in the north and in the south of the world [2]. Nonetheless the increasing demand from other healthcare organisations to use the platform led GHT to develop an open platform [3] that can therefore be adapted to the clinical and management of every healthcare centre that wants to use it. The large number of requests led us to open a virtual healthcare centre called Web Jolly, which collects the requests for teleconsultations that arrive sporadically from the farthest corners of the planet: requests for teleconsultations from Syria, from the refugee camps in Lebanon or from Pakistan and many other places, have been assigned to this geographically inexistent centre. There is great interest in this platform: in fact around 20 healthcare centres are asking to join the teleconsultation service.

At the beginning the service only provided cardiology teleconsultations, but within a few years, it has been able to offer teleconsultations for 18 different specialities (Fig. 9.2).

M. Bartolo (✉)
Telemedicine Unit, San Giovanni Hospital, Rome, Italy
e-mail: michelebartolo@gmail.com

F. Ferrari
University of Rome 'La Sapienza', Rome, Italy
e-mail: fabioferrari84@yahoo.it

© Springer International Publishing AG, part of Springer Nature 2018
M. Bartolo, F. Ferrari (eds.), *Multidisciplinary Teleconsultation in Developing Countries*, TELe-Health, https://doi.org/10.1007/978-3-319-72763-9_9

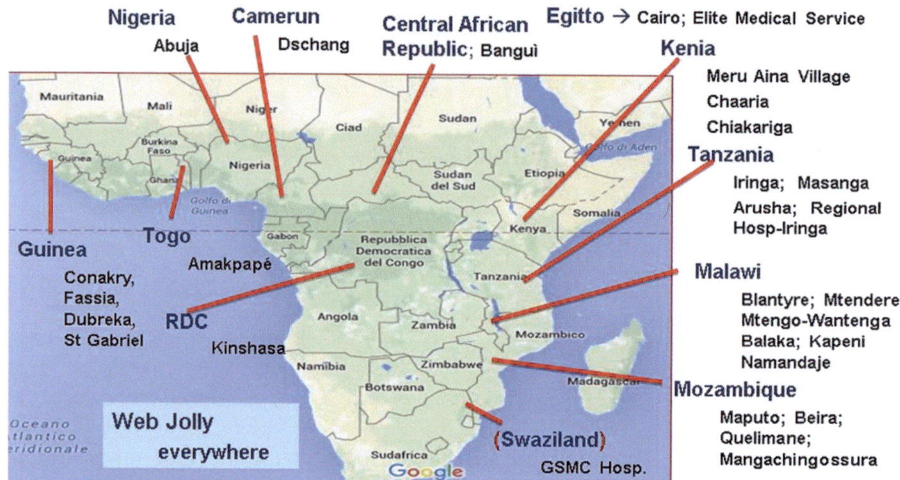

Fig. 9.1 GHT telemedicine centres in Africa

Today over 120 volunteer specialist doctors working in Italy and in Europe collaborate with GHT and guarantee answers over 1000 requests for teleconsultations a year.

Some of these specialists also take part in organising twice yearly training courses in the countries where GHT works, for the local staff [4]. Sometimes missions are carried out in order to explore the possibility of opening new centres and to supervise the ones that are already operative. These missions involve more people and means than up to a few years ago was even conceivable.

GHT has created a new way of cooperating, in which it is not only the doctors who travel but also the clinical information.

Actually teleconsultation is only the last step of a far more complex procedure that involves two different healthcare systems, a local one in Africa and a specialist one in Europe, and they communicate, sometimes in different languages, in order to agree on the best way to manage a certain clinical question. This all takes place at a distance of thousands of kilometres but almost in real time; almost, because the decision not to use real time was not only taken because of frequent connectivity issues in these areas [5], but above all in order to make it easier to organise the teleconsultations and all the work involved. The time to answer clinical questions varies depending on the number of specialists involved and the language requested. For cardiology, which has around 20 specialists, the answer is generally sent within an hour.

Fig. 9.2 List of medical specialities that can offer teleconsultation

- 1 Cardiology
- 2 Infectious diseases
- 3 Radiology
- 4 Internist physician
- 5 Pediatrician
- 6 Neurologist
- 7 Dermatologist
- 8 Nutritionist
- 9 Surgeon
- 10 Urologist
- 11 Ematology
- 12 Oculist
- 13 Gastroenterology
- 14 Vascular disease
- 15 Orthopedic
- 16 Burn
- 17 Endocrinology
- 18 Oncology

9.1 Steps Required for Setting Up a New Telemedicine Centre

All the steps dealt with in opening a new telemedicine centre are shown below.

9.1.1 Training for Local Staff

There is a whole chapter on training for local staff. All we want to say here is that training is essential if the remote centre is to work properly. Much of the training for medical staff concerns medical semiotics; knowing how to examine a patient makes it possible for the local health staff to provide the necessary information and limit the information that is not unnecessary. The software also has a section with specialist wizards, which asks the doctor the questions required for the specialisation selected.

The screenshots below are an example of the wizards used most often (Figs. 9.3 and 9.4).

The training for the technical staff involves explaining how to carry out maintenance, how the electromedical devices work and a considerable amount of time is spent on connectivity and local networks.

9.1.2 Remote Telemedicine Centre Instruments

With years of experience, we have identified the basic instruments for every healthcare centre that asks for teleconsultations. The instruments obviously vary from centre to centre. The minimum required is in any case a PC with an internet connection and with software that makes it possible to use the platform offline too, which is frequently found in Africa: this is one of the platform's most important features.

Dermatological data

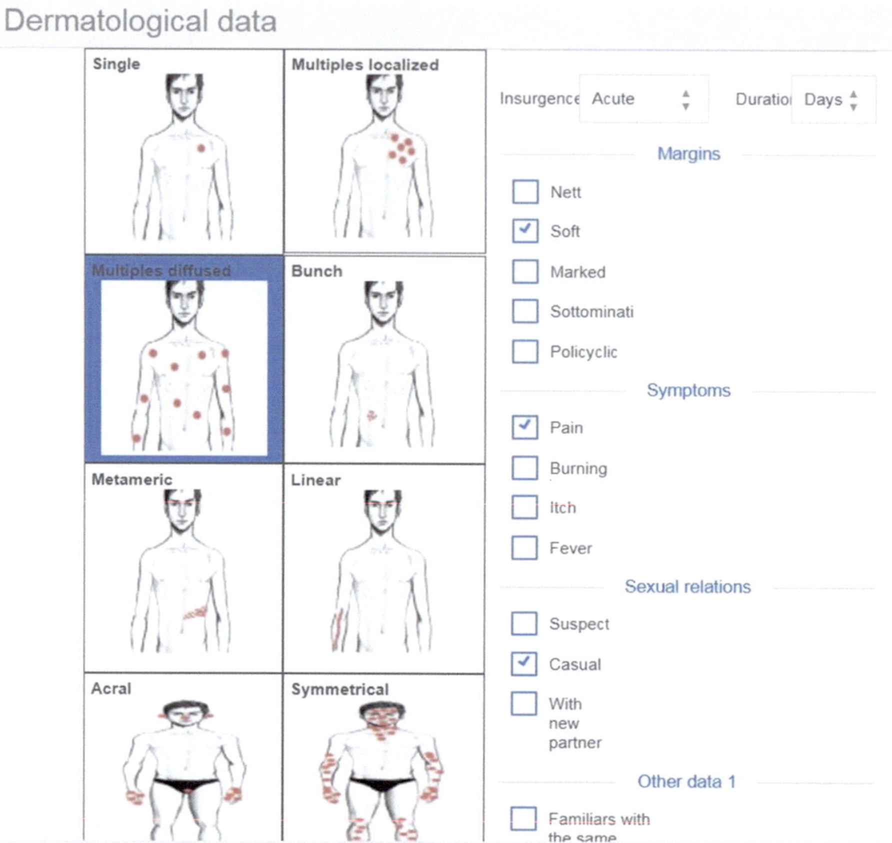

Fig. 9.3 Dermatological wizard examination

As well as a PC, a typical telemedicine centre also has an electrocardiograph that sends the ECG in pdf files, an oximeter and an HD webcam with a cable that is long enough to be able to take detailed photos of the patients. There is also a scanner for scanning X-rays or paper-based medical records provided by the patients (Fig. 9.5).

Some centres that have a neurology service also have an electroencephalograph that transmits the recording and the video of the recording. Very soon there will also be devices for transmitting retinography records, laryngoscopy records and scanners for pathological anatomy slides.

The telemedicine centres set up in the DREAM centres, thanks to the connection with the telemedicine platform with the DREAM Software [6], have enormous benefits. By simply entering the patients' ID, their personal information is uploaded, as well as their whole medical history with the vital parameters taken

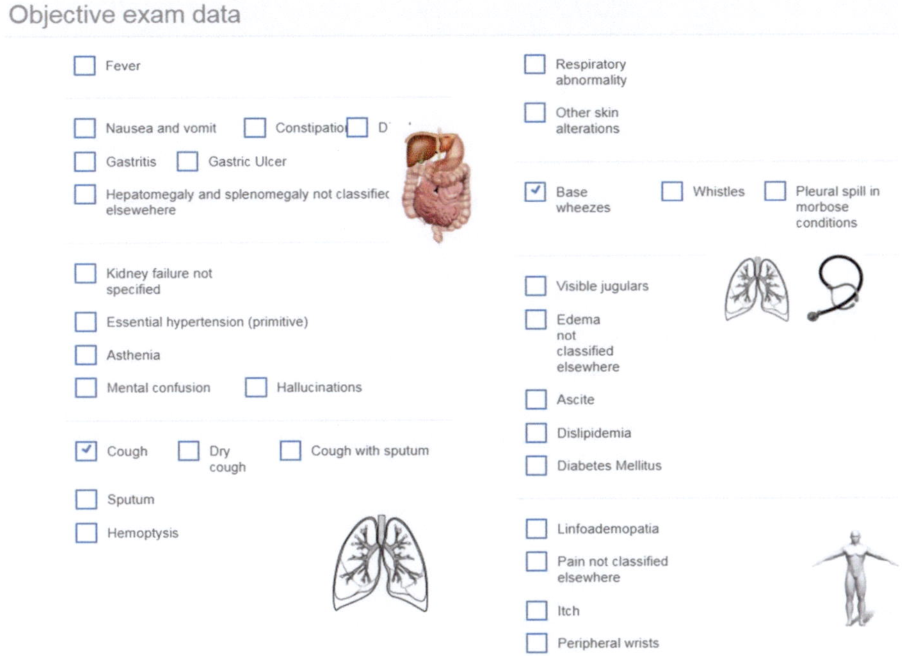

Fig. 9.4 Objective wizard examination

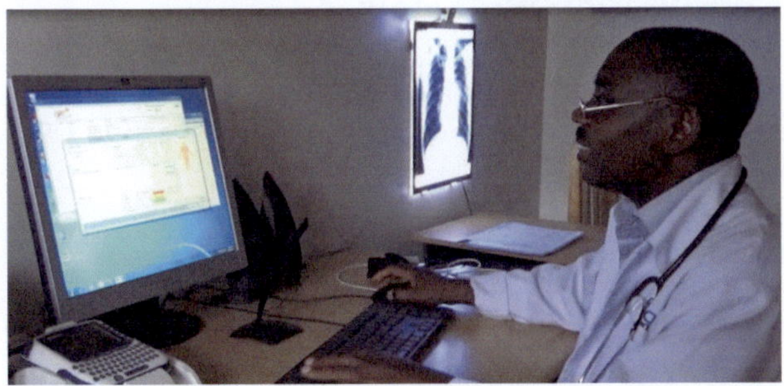

Fig. 9.5 Telemedicine centre in Arusha, Tanzania

during every examination, their blood tests, the therapy they are taking and even all the drugs present in the centre's pharmacy at that time. This last piece of information helps the doctor choose the therapy based on the drugs that are available in the healthcare centre (Fig. 9.6).

ID: IR005621							
Età	Sesso		Sieropositivo		Stadio AIDS	TARV	
5	M		HIV YES		4	TARV SI	

Data	CD4	CD8	CD4_CD8	CViral	Creat	GPT	GOT
2016-10-19					0.457	14.21	17.42
2016-01-13	36.05				0.594	6.112	36.28

Data	Leuco	Eritro	Hemo	Hema	VGM	HGM	CHGM	Plaq	LYM	MXD	NEUT	LYM2	MXD2	NEUT2
2016-10-19	6.4	4.42	12.0	44.2	100.0	27.1	27.1	619.0	54.6	7.9	37.5	3.54	0.54	2.44
2016-01-13	6.7	4.34	12.0	44.2	101.8	27.6	27.1	444.0	54.4	9.3	36.3	3.6	0.6	2.5

Data	BMI	TAmax	TAmin	FC	FR	TC
2017-04-10	14.85			125	25	36.2
Note,Diagnosi, Sintomi	Seen the boy has no complain, short appointment while wating fro TMC response this week. Dr.M					
2017-03-24	15.43			124	25	36.0
2017-03-24	15.43			124	25	36.0
Note,Diagnosi, Sintomi	Has no complains doing well nutrition is ok no cough chest clear Has high VL 86,305 Copies to send TMC to ct with Duovir N while awaiting for TMC ongoing counselling to the father on adherence and diet buy CTX 0.5 od/17days Dr.M					
2017-02-09	15.91			124	25	36.2

TARV				
Data	Stato	Motivo	Linea	Descrizione
Fri Apr 11 03:00:00 EAT 2014	TARV_SI		(3TC) + (AZT) + (NVP)	Duovir-N

Farmaci disponibili			
Nome Commerciale	Nome Composto	Posologia	Quantità
ABACAVIR SULFATE/LAMIVUDINE	ABC (600mg)	Compresse	1
ABACAVIR/LAMIVUDINE		Compresse	2
AMOXYCILLIN 250MG	Amoxicillin (250 mg)	Capsule	307
ATV/r	AZV (300 mg)	Compresse	861
Abacavir	ABC (300 mg)	Compresse	4304
Aciclovir- 200	Aciclovir (200 mg)	Compresse	1068
Albendazole	Albendazole (400mg)	Compresse	14421
Aluvia	LPV (200 mg) + RTV (50 mg)	Compresse	33165

Fig. 9.6 DREAM DB patient health report form

9.2 Teleconsultation WorkFlow

A summary of how every teleconsultation is organised is briefly illustrated in a 60-second video, which is available on the GHT website [7]. The following is a brief description of the workflow:

1. In a remote healthcare centre, a doctor or a nurse enters some of the patient's personal information on the platform and can describe the clinical case in a specific field.
2. If they want to, they can use either general or specialised wizards for an objective examination of the patient, which makes it possible to enter the symptoms and/or diagnosis with just one click.
3. They enter any medical records that are considered useful (images, electrocardiograms, blood tests, etc.).
4. They choose which department/departments to send the request for teleconsultation to, from the 18 specialities available.
5. They choose the degree of urgency (triage: white, green, yellow or red) and send the request via web. The centres that do not have a connection can carry out all these operations offline and then synchronise the data when they have access to internet again.
6. On the other side of the world, the doctors working within the speciality requested receive an alert by SMS or email. The first available doctor connects

to the platform with a PC, tablet or smartphone and reads the details of the request for teleconsultation and answers.

7. As soon as the doctor providing the service answers, the doctor requesting the service receives an SMS; they then connect to the platform and can see the diagnostic and therapeutic advice.

9.2.1 Helpdesk Services

In order to make sure that the teleconsultations work properly, there is a healthcare helpdesk, which consists mainly of nurses who use specific tools to supervise the timing and the way each teleconsultation is carried out. The healthcare helpdesk can intervene on either side of the teleconsultation, for either the doctor requesting or the doctor providing the service, and can close a request for teleconsultation or forward it to another speciality.

There is also a technological helpdesk that doctors requesting or providing teleconsultation can use for any technical issue.

9.3   A Model That Can Be Replicated

The increasing number of requests that reach us from healthcare centres all around the world indicates the strong interest in telemedicine.

Technology is essential for the platform to work properly, but technology alone is not enough. The strong point of GHT is that the model can also easily be replicated in other contexts. Sometimes, due to logistic issues, we have opened a remote centre and carried out the training in Rome, and the doctors who would be working in that centre took the equipment with them.

References

1. Global health telemedicine, this is how telemedicine is renewing cooperation between the north and the south of the world. http://www.sanita24.ilsole24ore.com/art/commenti/2014-12-03/global-health-telemedicine-cosi-121445.php?uuid=Abi3xQjK
2. Bartolo M. Sognando l'Africa in Sol Maggiore, Ediz Gangemi. Ch 15, 2014.
3. Frati D. Information Technology: risorsa o problema? Il pensiero scientifico editore, 2010.
4. Globalised healthcare, a pan-African training course in Maputo, by DREAM-GHT. http://www.sanita24.ilsole24ore.com/art/notizie-flash/2016-02-12/sanita-globalizzata-maputo-corso-formazione-panafricano-firmato-dream-ght-130319.php?uuid=ACuk02SC
5. Available on www.theguardian.com. https://www.theguardian.com/global-development-professionals-network/2014/jan/24/digital-divide-access-to-information-africa
6. Nucita A, Bernava G, Bartolo M, Peroni M, Palombi L. A global approach to the management of EMR (Electronic Medical Records) of patients with HIV/AIDS in sub-Saharan Africa: the experience of Dream Software. BMC J Med Inform Decis Mak. 2009:9(42).
7. http://www.ghtelemedicine.org/site/index.php/video

From on the Field Training to E-Learning 10

Fausto Ciccacci and Kingaru Shamsi

10.1 The Need for Training

Training is an essential part of both the DREAM and the GHT [1] programmes; every telemedicine programme has to be fully involved in training, in order to engage, motivate and teach the healthcare staff to use the technology.

The DREAM programme has been strongly committed to training local personnel and capacity building since it started in 2002. Similarly, GHT has also focused on training local staff as a key part of its programme. In 2016 alone the DREAM programme and GHT organised training sessions for more than 1000 health workers, medical doctors, medical officers, nurses, community social workers, biologists, laboratory technicians, etc.) in four countries (Mozambique, Malawi, Republic of Guinea and Tanzania). One of the biggest problems in Africa is the lack of health staff. There are not enough skilled medical doctors and nurses in most countries in Africa to cope with the huge number of patients. Most European countries have on average 1 medical doctor for 250 people, whereas in Africa the ratio is much lower: there is only 1 medical doctor for 10,000 people in the Republic of Guinea, which was recently badly affected by the Ebola infection; in Mozambique there is 1 doctor for 18,000 people, and in Malawi, one of the countries that is affected worst by HIV, the ratio is 1 doctor for 52,000 inhabitants [2]. The lack of skilled personnel is a critical issue for national health systems in Africa.

F. Ciccacci (✉)
'DREAM Program', Community of Sant'Egidio, Rome, Italy
e-mail: fausto.ciccacci@gmail.com

K. Shamsi
DREAM Program, Arusha, Tanzania
e-mail: kingarushamsi@gmail.com

© Springer International Publishing AG, part of Springer Nature 2018
M. Bartolo, F. Ferrari (eds.), *Multidisciplinary Teleconsultation in Developing Countries*, TELe-Health, https://doi.org/10.1007/978-3-319-72763-9_10

10.2 On the Field Training

The DREAM programme's training consists of several phases. Different settings can naturally modify the training agenda. Generally, the training activities concentrate on the implementation of good practices in health and the transfer of the lessons learnt into a real-life environment.

The training process can be described as follows:

- Assessment of training needs
- Setting training objectives
- Frontal training
- On-the-job training

As mentioned, the training can have different goals, but the aim is often to set up a health service or to improve a service that is already operative. In this case, the assessment of the needs is best done on the field, with visits carried out on-site. The training objectives have to be decided together with the health staff, in meetings held at different levels. During this phase it is very important to identify the right personnel to be trained, in order to achieve the specific objective (e.g. pharmacists and peer-to-peer educators if adherence to treatment has to be strengthened). Once the objectives have been decided, the training has to be organised with either traditional lessons or on-the-job sessions [3]. In most cases, a combination of the two is best. In traditional lessons it is important to provide enough time for case reports, role playing and real-life simulations. The lessons have to be as relevant to the trainees' experience as possible. In DREAM's experience, the choice of trainers is also very important. The right trainers have to be identified for the various needs and objectives. The DREAM programme sometimes organises training courses with professors from European or North American universities, but the courses often have local professors who are in charge of national health programmes. When it is important to train personnel on practical skills, it is best to have operational trainers such as clinical coordinators or experienced African colleagues.

The training method often involves "pan-African" training courses, which are a very important aspect of DREAM's vision and its mission [4]. The pan-African training courses have the great advantage of making the trainees feel they are part of the big health challenge for their continent. They are no longer isolated health workers, but they become leaders of change, sharing their mission with colleagues in other countries. This also greatly improves the quality of their work, as it strongly motivates staff. Motivation also is one of the training objectives in DREAM, since it makes the health workers feel part of the bigger challenge of caring for their people [5]. One of the key elements of DREAM's success is also excellence of care, which is not only a benefit for the patients but also for the health workers who operate in an efficient environment, making it possible for them to love their work [6].

10.3 Long-Distance Learning

Another aspect of the DREAM approach to training is e-learning and long-distance learning [7]. The DREAM model is based on the DREAM software, which is an excellent tool for managing and monitoring its healthcare activities, as fully described in Chap. 4. The DREAM software has also become an important instrument for e-learning as it is connected with a telemedicine platform that links together hundreds of specialists operating in Europe, who give their African colleagues second opinions [8]. This is first of all an opportunity for providing a high-quality service, but it also represents an important factor of capacity building for African personnel who receive a sort of "long-distance training on-the-job" [9].

In African healthcare centres, the services are often provided by non-medical health professionals (clinical officers, medical technicians, nurses, etc.) whose work is based on diagnostic/therapeutic algorithms developed by the ministries of health. The training they receive is generally based on these algorithms, and they often have trouble dealing with clinical situations for which there are no protocols.

Moreover, the doctors do not often have much experience with many of the pathologies that today are emerging in African countries and which on the other hand have been present in Europe for a long time: cardiovascular diseases, diabetes, dyslipidemias, cerebrovascular diseases, cancer, etc.

GHT's multidisciplinary teleconsultation service puts hundreds of European specialists in touch with African healthcare professionals, and it is a real form of "distance learning". The African staff can send requests for teleconsultations through the telemedicine platform, and they can also attach the results of medical tests including electrocardiogram recordings, X-rays, electroencephalograms, photographs of skin lesions, blood tests and also medical reports. They soon receive a diagnosis and therapeutic indications.

Over time the staff learn specialised skills with real training, which is like the training that medical students or postgraduate students receive in the hospital wards in Europe and the United States.

The frontal training sessions that regularly take place give the European (consultant) doctors and their African colleagues the chance to get to know each other. During these sessions, some of the cases that the African doctors have encountered during their "assisted" clinical practice can be discussed at length.

On the field training and e-learning are therefore not to be considered contradictory or as successive stages but as two parts that regularly interact and contribute to each other [10].

In order to better explain how the value of teleconsultation goes far beyond the individual clinical answer, here is an example of what happened in one of the first telemedicine centres, in Arusha, in Tanzania. After a residential course on cardiology held in 2008, we sent the centre an electrocardiograph, and during the first few months of work with the GHT platform, around 30 recordings a week were given medical reports. This trend was steady at the beginning, but after a few months, fewer and fewer recordings were sent and the trend then stabilised at just a few recordings a week. We thought there was a technical problem so we looked into why we were receiving so few requests for teleconsultations. The doctor's answer was very revealing: "By now I've learnt how to read the normal recordings or those with well-known electrocardiogram alterations, so I decided to only send the most complex recordings". This is a practical example of how teleconsultation is also continuous training.

References

1. http://it.radiovaticana.va/news/2017/03/18/telemedicina_nuova_frontiera_per_la_cooperazione_in_africa/1299116
2. World Bank data. Available at https://data.worldbank.org/indicator/SH.MED.PHYS.ZS
3. Frazis H, Loewenstein MA. On-the-Job-Training. Found Trends Microecon. 2007;2 (5):363–440. https://doi.org/10.1561/0700000008.
4. 2008 long life for Africa Leonardo International – pag. 107–113.
5. Manongi RN, Marchant TC, Bygbjerg C. Improving motivation among primary health care workers in Tanzania: a health worker perspective. Hum Resour Health. 2006;4:6. https://doi.org/10.1186/1478-4491-4-6.
6. Bonenberger M, Aikins M, Akweongo P, Wyss K. The effects of health worker motivation and job satisfaction on turnover intention in Ghana: a cross-sectional study. Hum Resour Health. 2014;**12**:43. https://doi.org/10.1186/1478-4491-12-43.
7. Cook DA, Levinson AJ, Garside S, Dupras DM, Erwin PJ, Montori VM. Internet-based learning in the health professions a meta-analysis. JAMA. 2008;300(10):1181–96. https://doi.org/10.1001/jama.300.10.1181.
8. Todd CS, Mills SJ, Innes AL. Electronic health, telemedicine, and new paradigms for training and care. Curr Opin HIV AIDS. 2017;12(5):475–87.
9. Edirippulige S, Armfield NR. Education and training to support the use of clinical telehealth: A review of the literature. J Telemed Telecare. 2017;23(2):273–282. First published date: February-17-2016. https://doi.org/10.1177/1357633X16632968.
10. http://www.askanews.it/cultura/2017/01/10/comunit%C3%A0-santegidio-arpa-insieme-per-la-telemedicina-no-profit-pn_20170110_00311/

GHT Activity Data

11

Fulvio Erba and Elena Cara

Since it started, GHT has provided 5512 teleconsultations covering various medical specialities. At the moment there are 29 centres in 12 African countries. Some requests for teleconsultations have reached us from areas of extreme hardship (Lebanese refugee camps, Syria). Cardiology is the specialisation that is requested most frequently, also because it is the specialisation that works best with telemedicine services. Other specialisations that are frequently requested include infectious diseases, dermatology, radiology, general medicine, neurology [1], orthopaedics and also plastic surgery, which was added because of all the burns from accidents that mainly involve children. Altogether we provide teleconsultation in 18 medical specialities, 89 African doctors are qualified to request teleconsultations and 121 European doctors answer these requests.

We could call this service "remote healthcare", which is a good way of describing a service that overcomes the question of distance.

Teleconsultation is a two-directional relationship between a doctor who has a request and one or more doctors who provide the answer.

The doctor asking for the teleconsultation makes a written request that may be accompanied by images, diagnostic tests, X-rays and medical records. The doctors providing the teleconsultation analyse all this information and write their diagnostic and or therapeutic suggestions on the same web-based platform.

In 2008 the first teleconsultations were requested using basic data transfer software. In 2013 GHT acquired a new data transfer system and installed client software in the centres requesting teleconsultations, which collects the data on a

F. Erba (✉)

Department of Clinical Sciences and Translational Medicine, University of Tor Vergata, Rome, Italy

e-mail: fulvio.erba@gmail.com

E. Cara

GHT Global Health Telemedicine, Rome, Italy

e-mail: elenacara13@gmail.com

© Springer International Publishing AG, part of Springer Nature 2018

M. Bartolo, F. Ferrari (eds.), *Multidisciplinary Teleconsultation in Developing Countries*, TELe-Health, https://doi.org/10.1007/978-3-319-72763-9_11

web platform. In view of the increase in the number of centres requesting teleconsultations, in February 2016 the whole data transfer system was redesigned and set up using a platform in collaboration with BS Innova. The technical details of the new platform are described in Chap. 12.

Taking into consideration all the requests for teleconsultations sent over the years with the different data transfer systems and platforms used by GHT, the total is 5512 requests for teleconsultations, directed to various specialities. For convenience, the following data and activities analysed refer exclusively to a period from February 2016 to 5 July 2017 and come from just the BS Innova platform, which is used by all our healthcare centres.

As of 5 July 2017, 29 healthcare centres in 12 African countries send requests for teleconsultations.

The Web Jolly, as described in Chap. 9, does not have a specific geographic location, but it collects requests for teleconsultations from different areas of extreme hardship (Lebanese refugee camps, Syria; etc.) (Table 11.1).

The centres in sub-Saharan Africa are in some of the poorest countries in the whole of Africa. Recently the Republic of Guinea and Sierra Leone were badly hit by the Ebola virus, which caused over 11,000 deaths [2]. For years there has been a war in the central-eastern areas of the Democratic Republic of Congo, which is between a civil war and a border war. The telemedicine service was set up in the Republic of Central Africa in 2015 during the civil war. Malawi is a country that risks famine because of the changes in seasonal rainfall and the impact of these changes on the country's mainly agricultural productivity. This is just a little information about the countries where the telemedicine service operates, and it clearly shows that service offered is even used in countries with the greatest hardships.

Looking at the characteristics of the software, one can see different user profiles that correspond to different aspects of the teleconsultation service. Table 11.2 shows the current profiles.

There are 89 "request doctors" (medical doctors or nurses), an average of 3 requesting doctors for every healthcare centre. In fact access has to be shared between more than one requesting doctor in the same centre in order to guarantee the continuity of the service. In any case, every requesting doctor can only see the teleconsultation that he requested, thus safeguarding the patients' privacy. Likewise, the answers provided for the centres can only be seen by the person who requested the teleconsultation.

There are 121 "response doctors", who belong to 18 specialities (see Table 9.1 in Chap. 9). Most of these doctors work in Italy, but there are also some responding doctors in France, Germany and Belgium. Every responding doctor can only see and answer the requests for teleconsultation that are sent to the speciality they belong to.

There are 8 "moderators" and they provide a healthcare helpdesk service. Most of the moderators are nurses, and they are coordinated by a doctor. Some of them work at the San Giovanni Hospital in Rome, which has signed an agreement to support the DREAM and telemedicine programme for Africa. Their job is to supervise the timing of every teleconsultation, but they can also intervene with

Table 11.1 List of healthcare centres requesting teleconsultations. DREAM® software. Authorised by ICT DREAM 2017

	Clinical centre	City	Country
1	DREAM_Crianca	Maputo	Mozambique
2	DREAM_Quelimane	Quelimane	Mozambique
3	DREAM_Polivalente	Beira	Mozambique
4	DREAM_Manga	Beira	Mozambique
5	DREAM_GSMH	Siteki	Swaziland
6	DREAM_Balaka	Balaka	Malawi
7	DREAM_Blantyre	Blantyre	Malawi
8	DREAM_Kapeni	Kapeni	Malawi
9	DREAM_Lilongwe	Lilongwe	Malawi
10	DREAM_Mtendere	Mtendere	Malawi
11	DREAM_Namandanje	Namandanje	Malawi
12	DREAM_ARUSHA	Arusha	Tanzania
13	DREAM_Iringa	Iringa	Tanzania
14	DREAM_Masanga	Masanga	Tanzania
15	IRH_Iringa	Iringa	Tanzania
16	DREAM_Meru	Meru	Kenya
17	DREAM_Chaaria	Chaaria	Kenya
18	DREAM_Chiakariga	Chiakariga	Kenya
19	BANGUI	Bangui	Central African Rep.
20	Amakpapè	Amakpapè	Togo
21	DREAM_Kinshasa	Kinshasa	Dem. Rep. of Congo
22	DREAM_Conakry	Conakry	Rep. of Guinea
23	DREAM_Dubreka	Conakry	Rep. of Guinea
24	DREAM_Fassia	Conakry	Rep. of Guinea
25	DREAM_St.Gabriel	Conakry	Rep. of Guinea
26	DREAM_Abuja	Abuja	Nigeria
27	DREAM_Dschang	Dschang	Cameroon
28	Elite Medical Services	Cairo	Egypt
29	WEB_JOLLY	Roma	Italy

the teleconsultation requests and answers. They intervene in an average of 35% of teleconsultations.

On www.ghtelemedicine.org, there is a function (Tableau Software) that provides a daily update of the requests and answers, and the information can be filtered using several different parameters. This provides an interactive and obviously anonymous visualisation of the teleconsultations, in terms of timing, origin, clinical specialisation and urgency (Fig. 11.1).

Teleconsultation activity data from February 2016 to 5 July 2017

Clicking on a country on the map selects the activities according to geographical areas or healthcare centres. This is important because it gives a real-time picture of

Table 11.2 User profiles. Authorised by GHT software (Global Health Telemedicine 2017)

Type	Description
REQUEST_DOCTOR	They can request teleconsultations for patients of the healthcare centre they are working in
RESPONSE_DOCTOR	They can only see and answer the requests for teleconsultations regarding their own speciality
MODERATOR	They check all the teleconsultation requests and answers. They can intervene by writing to both the doctors requesting and the doctors providing teleconsultations. They can close a request for teleconsultation at any time and can open it again or send it to another specialist
VIEWER	They check all the teleconsultation requests and answers but they cannot do anything
ADMINISTRATOR	This is the platform manager, for the creation and management of the users, of the healthcare centres, and of the identification of the specialities in which the doctors provide their services

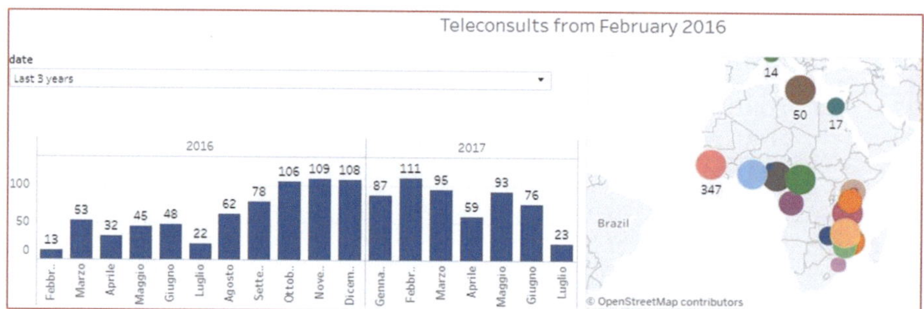

Fig. 11.1 Shows the data extracted from the GHT website regarding teleconsultation activities from February 2016 to 5 July 2017. Authorised by GHT website (Global Health Telemedicine 2017)

how the platform is being used, and it is therefore possible to intervene and solve the problems that affect the use of the teleconsultations [3].

Overall 1469 teleconsultations answers were sent (Fig. 11.2). Looking at the online statistics one can see that there were 1220 requests. This is due to the fact that many teleconsultations request the opinion of more than one medical speciality [4].

The platform is also designed to give the doctor requesting the teleconsultation and the doctor who sends the answer the opportunity to send several questions and answers if any aspects of the answer have to be explained or if it is necessary to go further into detail. In this case the teleconsultation turns into a chat, and this is one reason why there are more answers than questions.

The data show a difference in the use of the system and this depends on several factors. Connection problems in some areas are certainly one reason for this difference, but problems about the engagement and motivation of the local staff are another continuous reason.

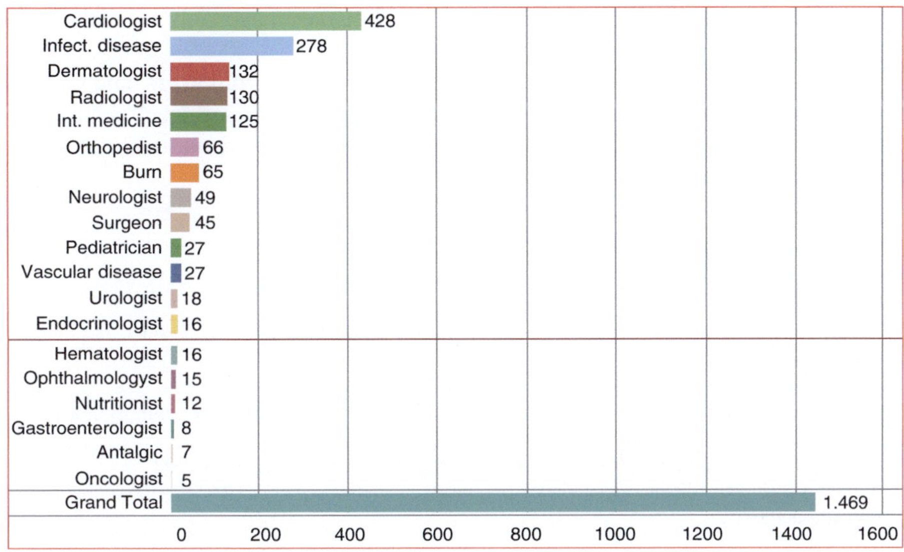

Fig. 11.2 Number of teleconsultation answers divided by category. Screenshot authorised by GHT website (Global Health Telemedicine 2017)

Dividing the requests for teleconsultations into medical specialities (Fig. 11.2) clearly shows that the speciality requested most is cardiology. Cardiology is a speciality that works well with teleconsultations, and it was the first speciality to be used. Every healthcare centre requesting teleconsultations has been provided with an electrocardiograph that communicates with the teleconsultation platform so it is possible to send electrocardiogram recordings to the specialists. Moreover the high number of cardiology teleconsultations requested and sent is also due to the screening that the DREAM programme is carrying out for hypertension and cardio-vascular diseases. These pathologies are increasing fast in Africa, as shown in Chap. 2, and a primary and secondary prevention campaign has been started for these diseases.

The second speciality in terms of frequency of requests is infectious diseases. The DREAM centres were initially set up as part of a programme for the prevention and treatment of HIV/AIDS, therefore paying particular attention to this infectious disease.

Other specialities (dermatology, radiology, general medicine) are required about once every four times with respect to the previous ones.

Over the years there has been an increase in the number of medical specialities provided, often because of the need to deal with requests that are not included in the initial agreement. The large number of requests for teleconsultation for people with burns, in particular children, led us to start the teleconsultation service for burns too. It is clear that radiology, as well as cardiology, is particularly important, since we work in countries where, although it is expensive, it is possible to have an X-ray done, but it is difficult to have it read.

There are some other medical specialities, but they have only recently been activated.

All the doctors who provide teleconsultation reports are volunteers, and GHT is increasing the number of specialists who want to offer their services for this new form of healthcare cooperation, which, even though it uses virtual technology, is absolutely concrete [5].

References

1. http://www.ghtelemedicine.org/site/index.php/rassegna-stampa/scientifica/165-abstract-sul-progetto-di-teleneurologia
2. WHO, Situation Report Ebola Virus Disease, 10 June 2016.
3. http://www.sanita24.ilsole24ore.com/art/europa-e-mondo/2017-03-09/reportage-sanita-si-globalizza-la-telemedicina-ponti-web-italia-e-malawi-124750.php?uuid=AEfFtsk
4. https://public.tableau.com/profile/ghtelemedicine#!/vizhome/GHT/Dashboard2
5. http://www.ghtelemedicine.org/site/index.php/rassegna-stampa/scientifica/162-premio-innovazione-digitale-sanita-2017

BS Innova Platform: Introduction, Framework and Technology

12

Giovanni Luca Soddu

12.1 Platform

BS Innova, in partnership with Global Health *Telemedicine and Community of S. Egidio*, has developed a services platform aimed to become a worldwide standard in the field of telehealth and telemedicine.

This platform allows physicians to analyse, diagnose and indicate treatments to patients in remote locations and provides access to medical competences quickly and efficiently. Platform's software includes a wide set of functionalities characterized by a "best of breed" web-based architecture.

The usage of this platform, with a "Software as a Service" (SaaS) model, is provided to different players in the field of healthcare systems: hospitals, major corporations for wellness programmes and non-profit health organizations. Since in general each player requires different specific modules, this platform includes "plug-in" components, in order to simplify the integration of additional modules developed by preselected technical partners to enrich the platform (e.g. any additional pathology wizards for teleconsulting).

Two different kinds of services are provided by this platform: *wellness services* and *teleconsultation services*.

The *wellness services* solution has been designed for the management of patients' clinical and behavioural data. The platform carries out important patient's health parameters and reports data directly to doctors or healthcare specialists. As this platform is being used in European countries, it will not be described further in this paper.

G. L. Soddu (✉)
BS INNOVA s.r.l., Telese Terme, Italy

BS INNOVA s.r.l., Roma, Italy
e-mail: g.soddu@bsinnova.it; gianluca.soddu@halcomict.it

© Springer International Publishing AG, part of Springer Nature 2018
M. Bartolo, F. Ferrari (eds.), *Multidisciplinary Teleconsultation in Developing Countries*, TELe-Health, https://doi.org/10.1007/978-3-319-72763-9_12

The *teleconsultation* solution (which is currently being used by 28 GHT centres) provides for management of patients' clinical and behavioural data, and it allows to manage the following:

- Guided insertion of requests for teleconsultation with "wizard" as to diseases with specific symptoms (i.e. cardiovascular, neurology, dermatology)
- Integration with medical devices for outcome analysis automatic loading (i.e. ECG, EEG, pictures, X-ray, electronic medical records for DREAM patients, lab results, ultrasound imaging, etc.)
- Automatic alerts to pools of specialists on the basis of the specialization/language
- Chat activation with specialists to advise on clinical insights and receive specific medical indication on care

12.1.1 Framework Architecture

The framework used to build this platform, developed by Applica (software house with HQ in Matera, Italy), is based on the *Spring Framework*, a standard in Java environment. This framework has been evaluated as the best one for managing the complexity of enterprise software applications, and, in the last few years, it has achieved a quality level hard to obtain by a from-scratch project.

In the picture below is shown the Spring Framework Architecture used to build the platform Fig. 12.1.

Framework's components are structured to obtain the top quality performances of the applications, which are standalones executable with an http server inside. This facilitates scalability, strong reduction in deployment time and, furthermore, the building of applications based on micro-services. The developed framework includes all the essential architectural patterns that a solid application must have (flux, dependency, MVC, [2] REST, etc.).

In order to avoid regression's issues and fully test the developed software, several build/test tools are used for unit and integration tests (Maven) [3], and also Continuous Integration (Jenkins) and UI test automation [4] processes are applied.

About the back-end application, all the previously mentioned technologies allow the development of a high-quality application. However, the increasing complexity of software and devices requires also a high-quality front-end application.

Therefore, also the front-end's application stack has been an important investment and has taken great effort in terms of innovation, research and development, architecture and design. To get the expected results, several innovative technologies have been used: ES6, HTML5/CSS3, Babel, Sass, React, Bower, Node, jQuery, Twitter Bootstrap and Material Design.

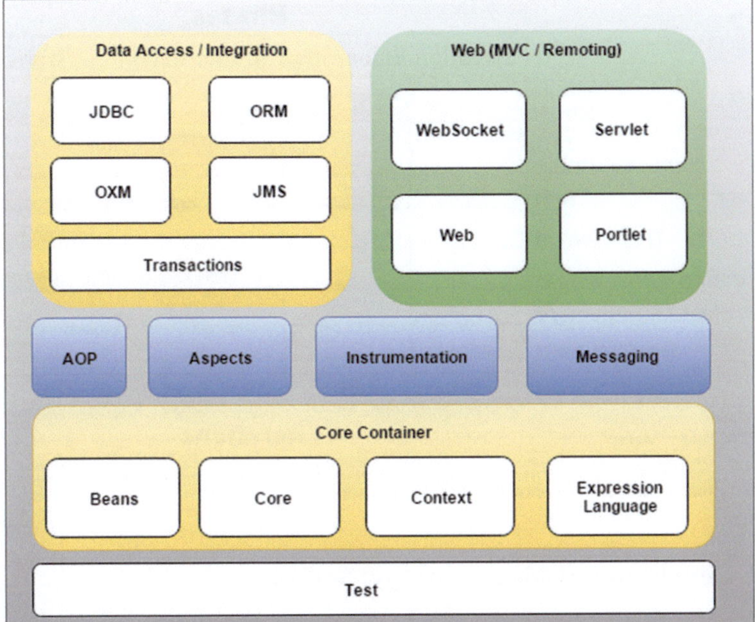

Fig. 12.1 Spring Framework architecture

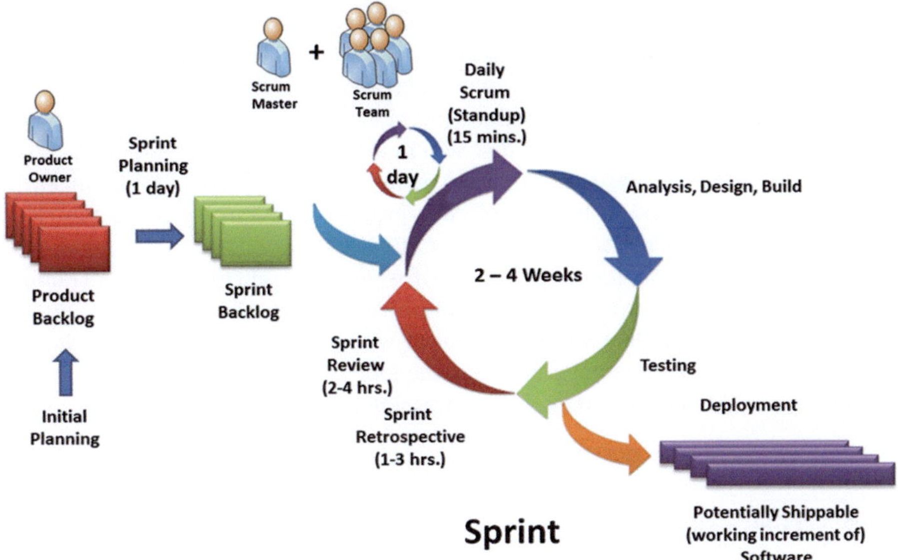

Fig. 12.2 Scrum methodology

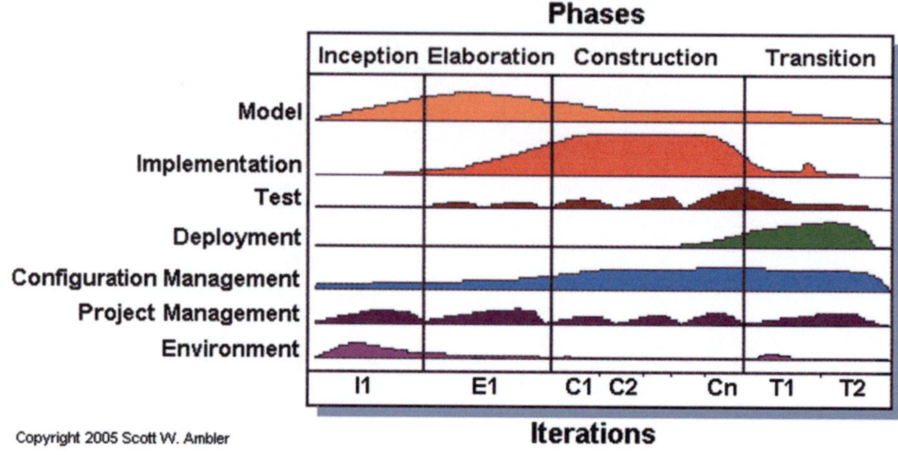

Fig. 12.3 Phases and activities of the Scrum method

12.1.2 Development Methodology: Scrum

The development of the platform leveraged the integration of the most remarkable benefits of the Agile [5] methodology (Scrum [6] based), with the advantage of well-defined analysis, design and documentation.

The applied processes have been tailored to manage the particular tasks and specific requirements of the project. In Fig. 12.2 the Scrum method is illustrated.

The main objective of the starting phase of *Inception* is to define its scope and to share description of the product before starting with development activities.

The next phase, *Elaboration*, defines the global system's structure. This phase includes the domain analysis and a first step in the architecture development.

In the third phase, *Construction*, "work items" are selected for development, in order to be implemented at the end of each process iteration. By doing this, it is possible to manage incremental/iterative improvements.

In the last phase, *Transition*, developed software is released to the client. Training and beta testing activities are conducted in order to verify and validate the system while assessing the product's full compliance with the requirements established in phase I; if this condition is not confirmed, the loop is repeated.

In Fig. 12.3 the four different phases are shown, with the related activities.

12.2   Technology

The software design process was focused on a required specific system capability: to provide the service in remote locations (Africa) where Internet connectivity is an issue. Several considerations have been made on the feasibility of the web platform development, where all data are managed centrally and must be accessible to all locations, irrespective of the Internet connectivity.

The chosen solution was to install the software as an executable in each machine and allow it to synchronize on demand with the central server as soon as the connectivity is available.

Several solutions were then considered in relation with the kind of application to be developed: a desktop application or another kind of solution? The main issue lay with the fact that the complexity and amount of data managed by the software were computationally too heavy to be managed by a clone application on a desktop platform.

The development of a new technological and architectural web solution allowed the platform to operate also in an *off-line mode*. The provided solution exploits the usage of the portable web server "Jetty"; this server allows the platform to run on a local machine through an executable, which starts the web server Jetty and, by doing so, runs locally the web platform (in a local configuration mode).

This solution eliminates this complexity and avoids having to manage two different applications for the web and the local system. The local application then stores locally all data and sends them to the central system when the connectivity is available (synchronization process).

Other issues that have been addressed:

- How to ensure that the central destination system (master) will receive all the correct and proper data sent by the local machines?
- How to ensure that possible loss of connectivity won't impact the data transfer?
- How to manage potential conflicts, in terms of changes done by both the local and the central systems with respect to the same teleconsultation?

To address these points, a new set of algorithms was selected, as described in the following workflow (Fig. 12.4).

In this diagram, the source (e.g. the local system) requires the destination (central system) to start the data synchronization. The built procedure can be described by the following steps:

Step 1 Source starts synchronization session with destination.

During this step, the source starts the communication with the destination. The connection phase between the source and destination is called *synchronization session*.

Step 2 Destination prepares a response and sends knowledge.

As mentioned before, each response stores its own unique knowledge, and knowledge stored in the destination is sent back to the source.

Step 3 Destination knowledge is used to determine the changes to be made.

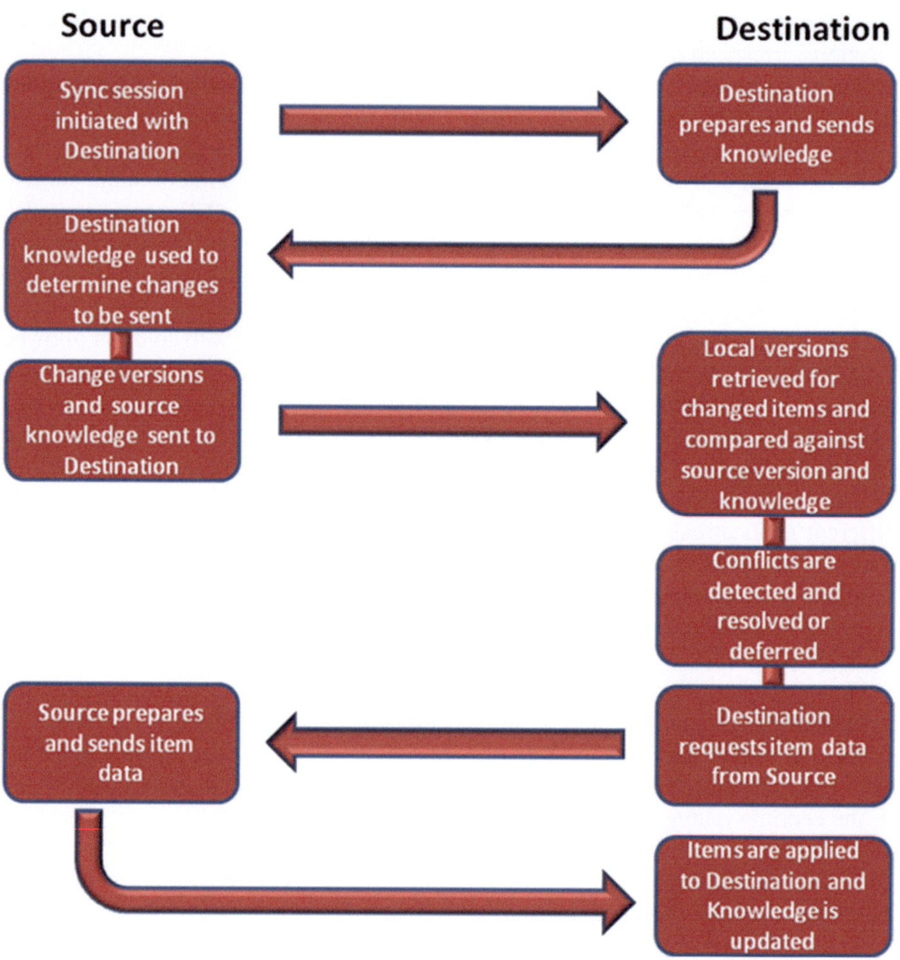

Fig. 12.4 Communication algorithm's outline

The source, as soon as data are received, compares them with the related local data, in order to establish which elements the destination doesn't know. It is important to note that the versions that are sent are not the real elements, but they are just, for every element, a summary of the place where the last modification was made.

Step 4 Versions of the changes and knowledge of the source are sent to the destination.

Once the source has prepared the list of the requested change versions, those are sent to the destination.

Step 5 Versions of changes made in local are extracted and compared with the versions and knowledge of the source.

The destination uses those versions to prepare a list of elements that the source has to send. The destination uses also this information to detect conflicts.

Step 6 Conflicts are detected, resolved or deferred.

A conflict is detected when the version of a change in a reply does not contain the knowledge of the other. Basically, a conflict occurs if a change is applied to the same element on two replies between synchronization sessions. Specifically, conflicts occur when the knowledge of the source does not include the version of destination for any specific element (supposing destination knowledge does not include any of the sent source versions).

If the version is included in the destination knowledge, the change is considered as obsolete. Replies, using a data merging approach, can implement several criteria for the resolution of conflicting elements.

12.2.1 Interface Architecture

As already specified the platform has a web application interface, which was built using Spring MVC technology. This technology allows the creation of an environment where it is possible to split out several roles of interface design and preparation with real data.

12.2.2 Back-End Architecture

Having used Spring MVC as server side interface, REST services have been built by exploiting the Spring Framework to provide support for the dependency injection, for annotations on controllers, rest controllers, etc.

12.2.3 Security

Security has also been based on the Spring Security framework; the platform's domain is based on the communication protocol for secure communication *HTTPS*. For the registration process, the new user has to follow a precise authentication procedure, with a password and specific encryption. After submitting a request for registration and its subsequent approval, an e-mail is sent to the new user requesting for confirmation of registration. Furthermore, to enhance the security standard of the platform, the OWIN encryption has been developed; this encryption module defines a standard interface between .NET web servers and web applications.

12.2.4 Platform Technical Specifications

The platform has been built with the purpose to design an architecture characterized by the following features:

- Availability
- Performance
- Reliability
- Maintainability
- Scalability

In order to build the platform with the mentioned characteristics, Java development language has been selected on the grounds that it is the most suitable language to verify them and, also, the most common language used for enterprise SaaS solutions. The main reasons are:

- It is a compiled language (this feature increases performance as compared to interpreted language).
- It is a typed language (this quality reduces the chance of error and increases the system's performance).
- It allows a better organization of the code.
- It has an advanced debugger.
- It has an advanced profiler (profiling allows to obtain a list of the information related to the code's execution performances; this is greatly useful to better understand and solve code performance quality problems and inefficiencies).
- Better web services management.
- Better deployment environment.
- Higher-quality framework (Hibernate, Apache Commons).

12.2.5 Modularity

The core module is developed throughout the implementation of a set of functionalities capable to respond to basic requirements. Besides the core module and its standard functionalities, add-on modules can be integrated into the platform through a standard layer; these functionalities are able to cover specific pathologies. This means that anyone, following the development standard defined by BS Innova and implementing this integration layer, is able to develop other modules for different, specific therapeutic areas; this allows the platform to have an efficient modular structure.

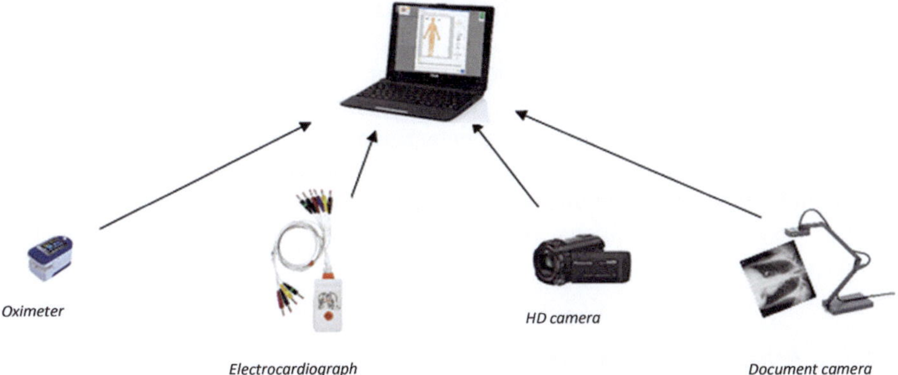

Fig. 12.5 Teleconsultation standard kit

12.2.6 Medical Device Integration

With the teleconsultation service, the platform was thought to be the core of a system of different medical devices, with the task to collect and send, through the teleconsultation module, the acquired patient's health parameters. As of today, the kit used in the Africa centres is equipped with the following devices (Fig. 12.5):

- Oximeter (*LifeMed*)
- Electrocardiograph BLE (*Cardioline Touch ECG*)
- HD camera
- Document camera (*IPEVO*)

All devices are characterized by their highly user-friendly interface and their simple installation procedure; the whole system, in the end, is able to collect several parameters and information about the patient's health, such as oxygen saturation, heart rate, ECG, EEG and X-ray, besides being able to acquire other data such as pictures, slabs and videos.

The integration between the different devices' software and the platform is supplied by the possibility to load and send different types of files on the platform. By doing this, the requesting doctor is able to attach different files to the request module, enhancing the detail and quality of information in the request module.

At the moment, BS Innova is considering to widen the set of medical devices in order to integrate to the platform different systems capable to analyse more extended and complex therapeutic areas.

12.2.7 Tele-Video and Tele-Chat Consultations

The platform delivers asynchronous teleconsultations, by this meaning that between the request and the response, between the doctors, there is no real-time interaction. By now BS Innova is starting to implement additional functionalities in order to deliver, in the future, new services such as video consultation and real-time chat consultation; these future applications will increase the efficiency and the quickness of response in teleconsultations, thus allowing a much faster and clearer interaction between the request and the response.

12.2.8 Additional Features

Other platform's technical features include usability and multilanguage features. Usability was one of the most important properties taken into consideration for the development of the software; as a result, the platform exhibits a user-friendly interface and configuration procedure. As a matter of fact, many non-profit organizations have already gained access to the platform rapidly and easily as the software is effectively "self-explaining" and consists in a plug and play installation of some standard devices.

The platform also includes a multilanguage feature which performs an automatic translation of the request and response module into four different European languages, so both the requesting and the responding doctor can write in their own native (or more fluent) languages without any concern.

Activity data on platform usage are reported in detail in Chap. 11.

References

1. Norris AC. Essential of telemedicine and telecare. Chichester: Wiley; 2001.
2. Gupta P, et al. MVC design pattern for the multi framework distributed applications using XML, spring and struts framework. Int J Comput Sci Eng. 2010;02(04):1047–51.
3. Paschke A. OntoMaven: maven-based ontology development and management of distributed ontology repositories. In: Proceedings of the 9th International Workshop on Semantic Web Enabled Software Engineering (SWESE 2013); 2013.
4. Peleska J, Siegel M. Test automation of safety-critical reactive systems. S Afr Comput J. 1997;19:53–77.
5. Livermore JA. Factors that significantly impact the implementation of an agile software development methodology. J Softw. 2008;3(4):31–6.
6. Cardozo E, Araújo Neto B, Barza A, França C, da Silvia F. SCRUM and productivity in software projects: a systematic literature review. In: 14th International conference on evaluation and assessment in software engineering; 2010. p. 1–4.

Part IV

The Technology in Africa

The Digital Divide

13

M. Peroni and Michelangelo Bartolo

The digital divide is the gap between those who can access digital information and use it and those who are excluded, whether partially or totally. The word digital refers to the numerical representation of information for data processing or for telecommunications, and digital divide refers, rather than to the gap in the use of the instruments that provide this information, to the gap regarding the development of interconnection data networks, in other words, the Internet.

The definition appeared during the 1990s in the United States and became popular after it was used publically by the American President Clinton [1] and by the Vice President Al Gore, to indicate the gap between some areas of the United States that did not have access to the Internet and others that did, while the network was developing in the United States. This expression is now commonly used, not only within various national contexts but also in a global context, to indicate the gap in between rich and poor countries in their use of the Internet.

In 2000 at the World Economic Forum in Davos, a special committee, sponsored by several companies working with telecommunication technologies, was set up in order to close the digital divide. Since then many studies have been carried out to identify the causes of this gap and find solutions. The factors involved are economic reasons, lack of infrastructures and computer illiteracy. However today even though this gap still exists, the development of the network is taking place at an astonishing rate. In 2000, regarding the development of the Internet in the United States in that period, Jeffrey I. Cole (Director of the UCLA Center for Communication Policy) pointed out that "The Internet has become the fastest growing electronic technology in world history. In the United States, for example, after electricity became publicly

M. Peroni (✉)
'DREAM Program', Community of Sant'Egidio, Rome, Italy
e-mail: dream@santegidio.org

M. Bartolo
Telemedicine Unit, San Giovanni Hospital, Rome, Italy
e-mail: michelebartolo@gmail.com

© Springer International Publishing AG, part of Springer Nature 2018
M. Bartolo, F. Ferrari (eds.), *Multidisciplinary Teleconsultation in Developing Countries*, TELe-Health, https://doi.org/10.1007/978-3-319-72763-9_13

available, 46 years passed before 30% of American homes were wired; 38 years passed before the telephone reached 30% of U.S. households, and 17 years for television. The Internet required only seven years to reach 30% of American households" [2]. In fact today the impact of this observation can be applied to the whole world.

The speed of the growth of the Internet has some paradoxical aspects, which we can see particularly in Africa, where telephone services and the Internet can reach the population more easily than electricity in their homes. For example, there was a remote village in a rural area of Angola, where people lived in huts and the nearest electric power lines and an aqueduct were miles away. However the village chief had a mobile phone, not a smart phone, but an old model, whose battery lasted for days without having to be charged and in any case it was easy to charge with a small solar panel.

The cost of supplying electric power along copper cables has not decreased over the years, whereas thanks to the development of increasingly effective technologies, transmitting data with radio waves, that is, wireless transmission, is becoming less and less expensive. One could say that the cost of copper is measured in metres and the cost of radio transmission is measured in kilometres.

This is all particularly true for Africa, where the Internet developed differently to the way it developed in, for example, Italy.

In fact in Italy, during the years when the Internet was first being developed, there was a widespread network of copper telephone lines, so the distribution of the Internet to people's homes initially took advantage of these lines, first with modems using telephone lines, then with ADSL and then with FTTC (Fibre to the Cabinet), where the optic fibre cable is run from the telephone exchange to the street cabinets and the copper cable goes from the street cabinet to the home. In Africa, where the cable telephone network was practically non-existent, it was much more practical to invest directly in wireless technology.

However, these examples only show what happens at the end of the network, the section that reaches the user, the so-called last mile. Regarding the question of the digital divide in Africa or in less developed countries in general, another important factor is the capacity of the providers of the last mile to connect with the main backbone, that is, the worldwide networks that are the heart of the Internet.

When in 2002 work started on the Internet in Africa, in particular Mozambique, with the DREAM programme, the only way to transmit data was through a telephone modem. Attempting to provide assistance from Italy through the Internet was unthinkable because the cost would have been exorbitant. The connection to the international backbone took place exclusively via satellite, and because of the high cost of this service, the economically viable contracts for connections that were offered had such a high number of people sharing the connection at the same time that only low-speed operations were possible. So at the beginning we had to devise procedures for sending additional data with procedures for sending the messages again if necessary. Obviously the availability of only a low bandwidth made it impossible to have video conferences or provide remote assistance. At the beginning a satellite Internet connection was only necessary for telecommunication companies,

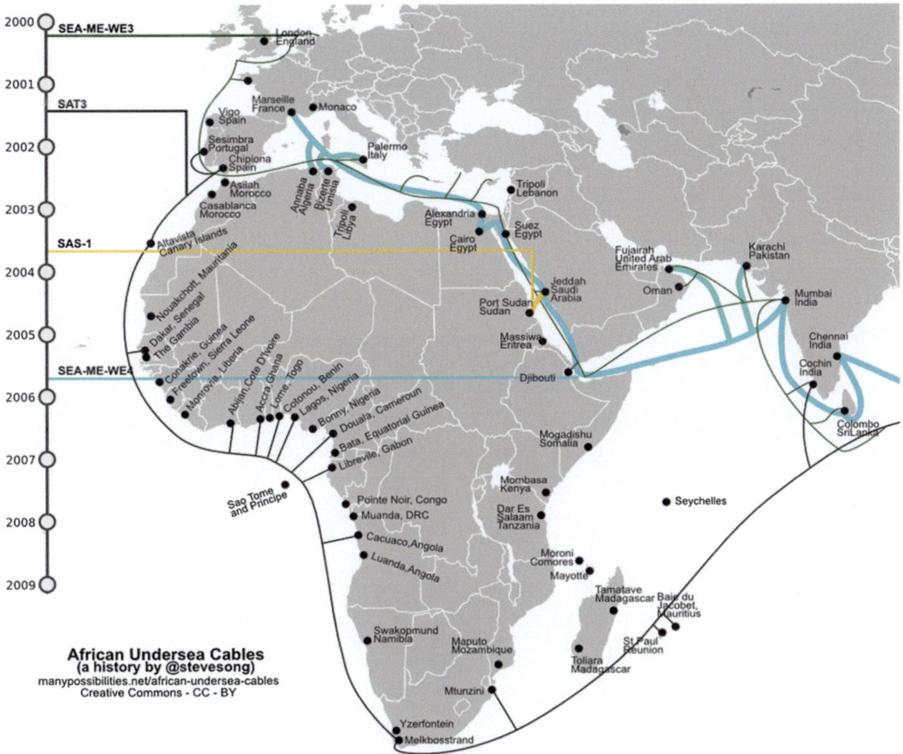

Fig. 13.1   African undersea cable in 2009

and it required large-scale installations and antennas. In the following years, there was an increase in the number of satellite providers offering Internet connections, if not for home use, at least for businesses, also, for example, for hospitals and health centres, and in contexts like the DREAM programme. At first almost all the centres were connected to the Internet this way, but as soon as it was possible, we started using local providers which, since they were connected to the international backbones with optic fibre cables, offered fast connections at a good price. In fact for satellite connections, the providers had to make large investments, in order to purchase, install and maintain the antennas and equipment needed for receiving and transmitting data via satellite. However, the fact that it was possible to connect to the international backbones with optic fibre cables brought the prices down, and consequently there was an increase in the offer, with considerable advantages for the final user, which, together with a reduction in costs, also led to a remarkable improvement in the service.

Between 2009 and 2013, at least eight large optic fibre backbones were set up around Africa, and they reached all the coastal countries (Fig. 13.1) [3]. The optic

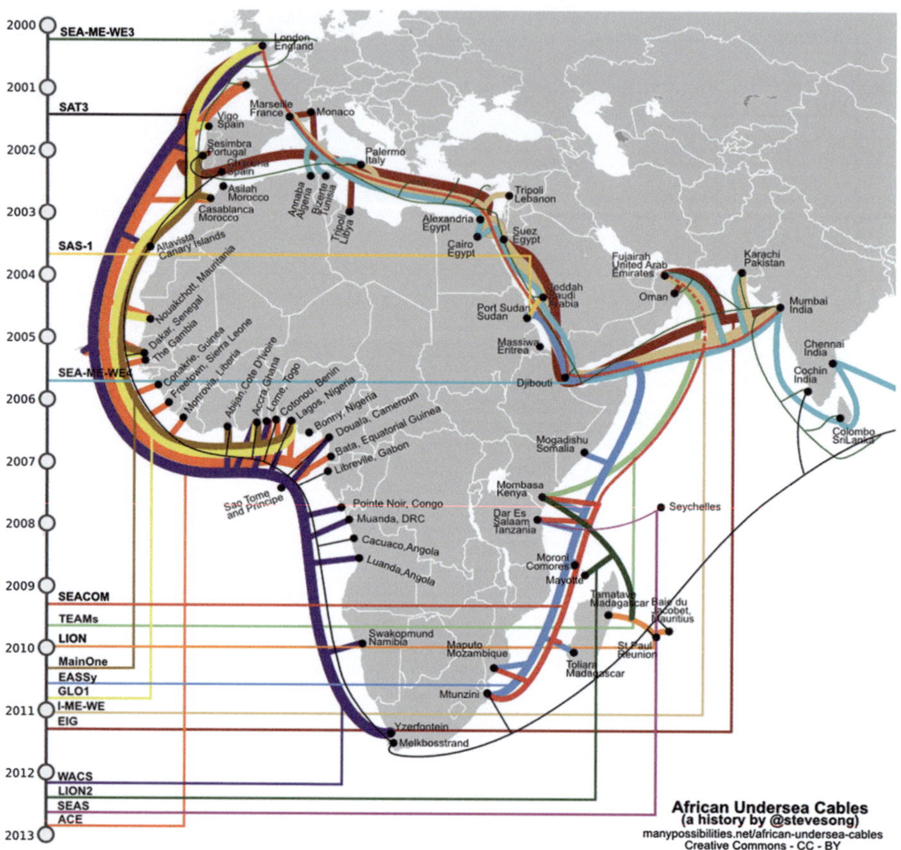

Fig. 13.2 African undersea cable in 2013

fibre branches then spread inland. Obviously laying the optic fibre cables under the sea did not mean that the country they were in front of could automatically have Internet connections. It was years, for example, before the optic fibre cable that had been laid under the sea off the Guinea-Conakry coast was provided with branches leading to the mainland.

However as soon as the connection was made, it was easy to see the benefits, and we could stop using the satellite connection in Conakry for one of our DREAM centres and rely on local providers, which had optic fibre connections and offered better results (Fig. 13.2).

The latest submarine lines that surround Africa today offer a much greater bandwidth than first ones that were laid. For example, the SAT3 (South Atlantic 3/West Africa Submarine Cable), which has been in service since 2001, can support a data flow of up to 800 Gbps, whereas the WACS (West Africa Cable System), which came into service 11 years later, supports a flow of 14.5 Tbps, and this is 18 times more, as though 18 new cables had been laid, instead of one.

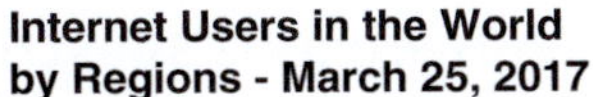

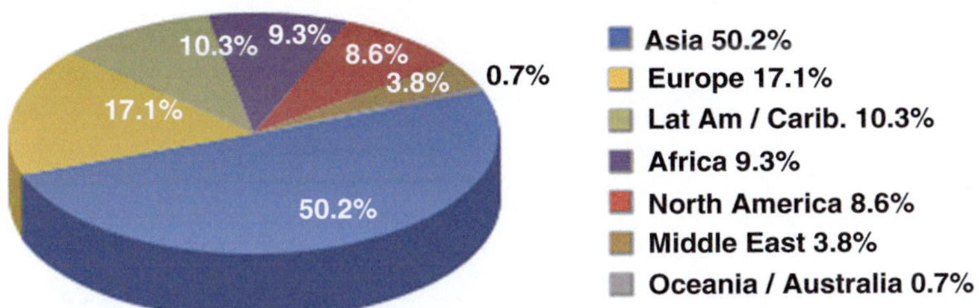

Source: Internet World Stats - www.internetworldstats.com/stats.htm
Basis: 3,731,973,423 Internet users on March 31, 2017
Copyright © 2017, Miniwatts Marketing Group

WORLD INTERNET USAGE AND POPULATION STATISTICS JUNE 30, 2017 - Update						
World Regions	Population (2017 Est.)	Population % of World	Internet Users 30 June 2017	Penetration Rate (% Pop.)	Growth 2000-2017	Internet Users %
Africa	1,246,504,865	16.6 %	388,376,491	31.2 %	8,503.1%	10.0 %
Asia	4,148,177,672	55.2 %	1,938,075,631	46.7 %	1,595.5%	49.7 %
Europe	822,710,362	10.9 %	659,634,487	80.2 %	527.6%	17.0 %
Latin America / Caribbean	647,604,645	8.6 %	404,269,163	62.4 %	2,137.4%	10.4 %
Middle East	250,327,574	3.3 %	146,972,123	58.7 %	4,374.3%	3.8 %
North America	363,224,006	4.8 %	320,059,368	88.1 %	196.1%	8.2 %
Oceania / Australia	40,479,846	0.5 %	28,180,356	69.6 %	269.8%	0.7 %
WORLD TOTAL	7,519,028,970	100.0 %	3,885,567,619	51.7 %	976.4%	100.0 %
NOTES: (1) Internet Usage and World Population Statistics updated as of June 30, 2017. (2) CLICK on each world region name for detailed regional usage information. (3) Demographic (Population) numbers are based on data from the United Nations Population Division. (4) Internet usage information comes from data published by Nielsen Online, by ITU, the International Telecommunications Union, by GfK, by local ICT Regulators and other reliable sources. (5) For definitions, navigation help and disclaimers, please refer to the Website Surfing Guide. (6) Information from this site may be cited, giving the due credit and placing a link back to www.internetworldstats.com. Copyright © 2017, Miniwatts Marketing Group. All rights reserved worldwide.						

Fig. 13.3 World Internet usage and population Statistics, 2017. www.internetworldstats.com

Another paradox of this rapid development is that Africa, as a continent, has the lowest percentage of Internet users throughout its population, whereas the number of people using the Internet in Africa is already higher than the number of people using the Internet in North America, which has the highest percentage of Internet users worldwide (Fig. 13.3).

(http://www.internetworldstats.com/stats.htm) [4].

The following is an analysis of the growth of voice and data telecommunications over the last decade.

The first aspect to take into consideration is the increase in mobile phone subscriptions, which is very important for transmitting data over the last mile, in that the data network can easily be spread on the mobile phone network pylons.

Regarding the percentage increase, that is, how many out of every 100 people have a mobile phone subscription, one can see that the gap has become progressively

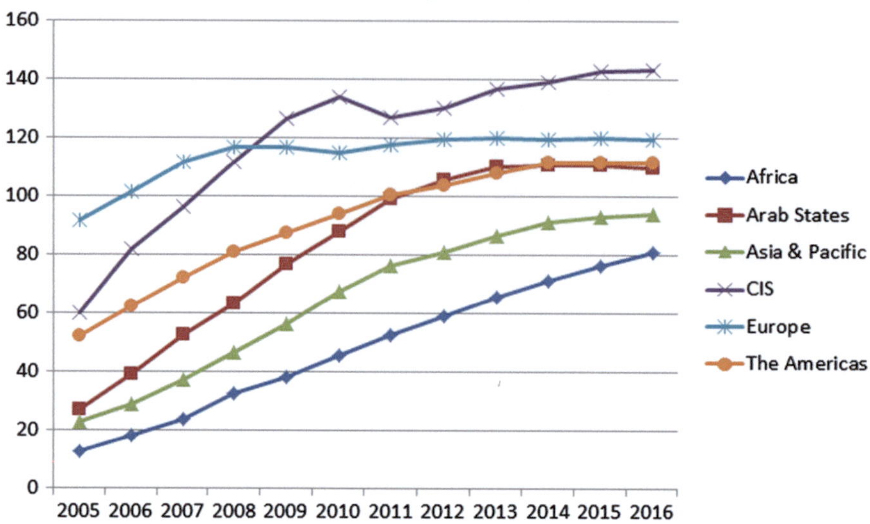

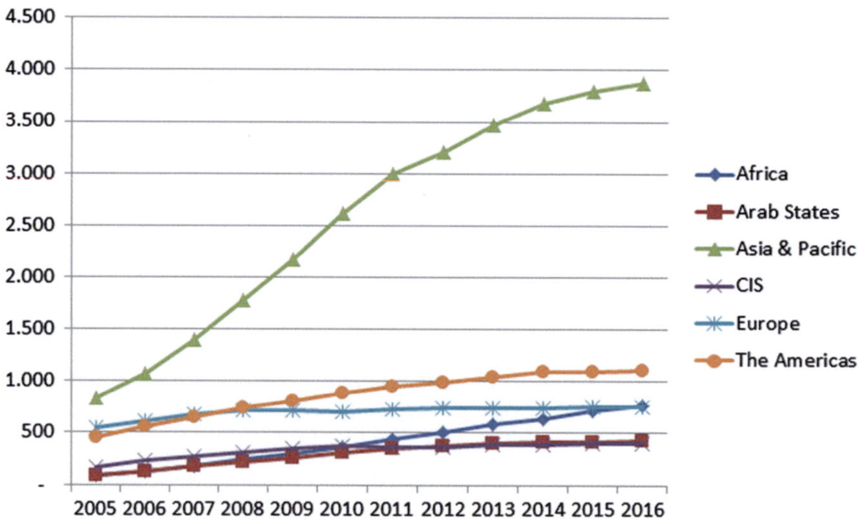

Fig. 13.4 My graphics, data from www.itu.int (http://www.itu.int/en/ITU-D/Statistics/Pages/stat/default.aspx)

narrower over the years, but if one looks at the increase in absolute terms, surprisingly enough Africa now has just as many mobile phone subscriptions as Europe (Fig. 13.4).

If one considers how many people use mobile Internet, one can see that the increase has taken place even faster, and even though the percentage is lower than in the rest of the world, the growth curve for Africa has been extremely steep in the last few years, which is a sign of exponential growth (Figs. 13.5 and 13.6).

http://www.itu.int/en/ITU-D/Statistics/Pages/stat/default.aspx

Finally, in 2002 less than 1 out of 100 people in Africa used the Internet compared to almost 21% of the people in Europe. Fourteen years later, in 2016, the percentage increased 4 times to 80% in Europe, whereas in Africa it increased 25 times (Figs. 13.7 and 13.8).

In conclusion, above all in analysing the trend of the increase over the last few years, although there is still a digital divide, above all between Africa and the rest of the world, one can see a rapid increase in the use of the Internet that is very encouraging for the near future.

DREAM's telemonitoring services and above all the multi-speciality Global Health Telemedicine teleconsultation services would not have been possible without this fast increase in internet connectivity in Africa.

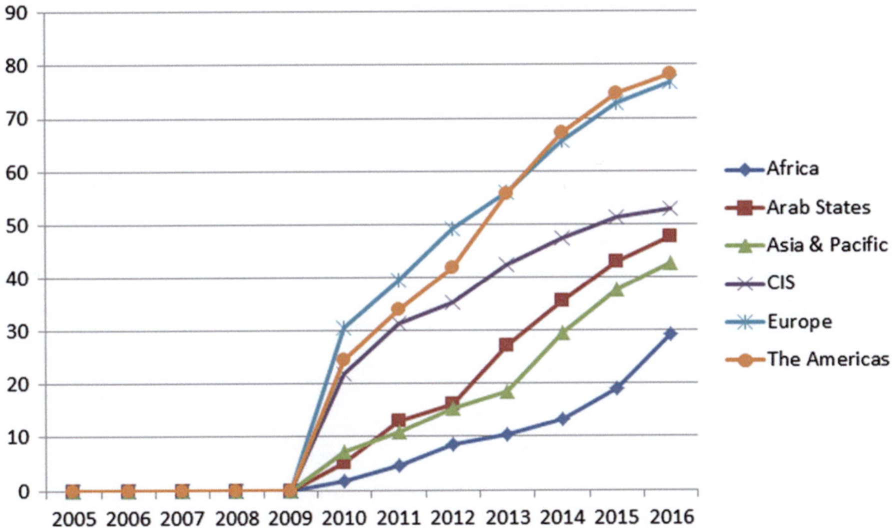

Fig. 13.5 Active mobile-broadband subscriptions (%). My graphics, data from www.itu.int (http://www.itu.int/en/ITU-D/Statistics/Pages/stat/default.aspx)

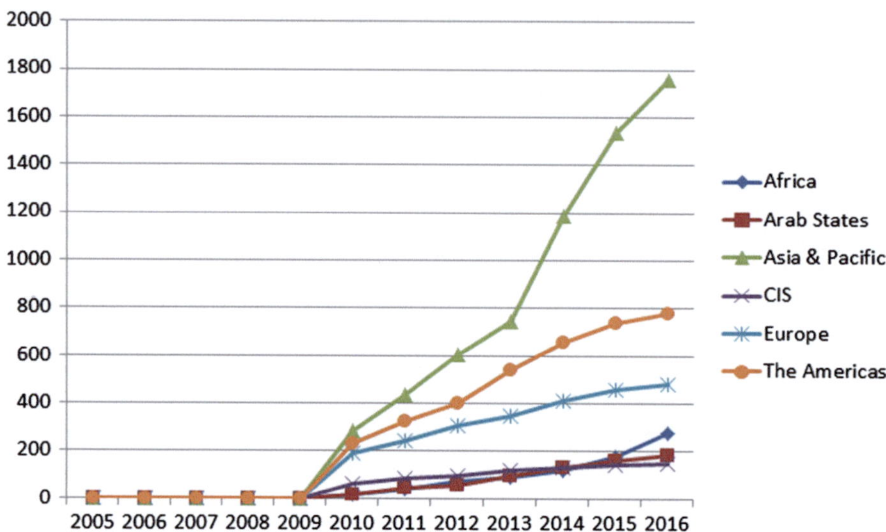

Fig. 13.6 Active mobile-broadband subscriptions (millions). My graphics, data from www.itu.int (http://www.itu.int/en/ITU-D/Statistics/Pages/stat/default.aspx)

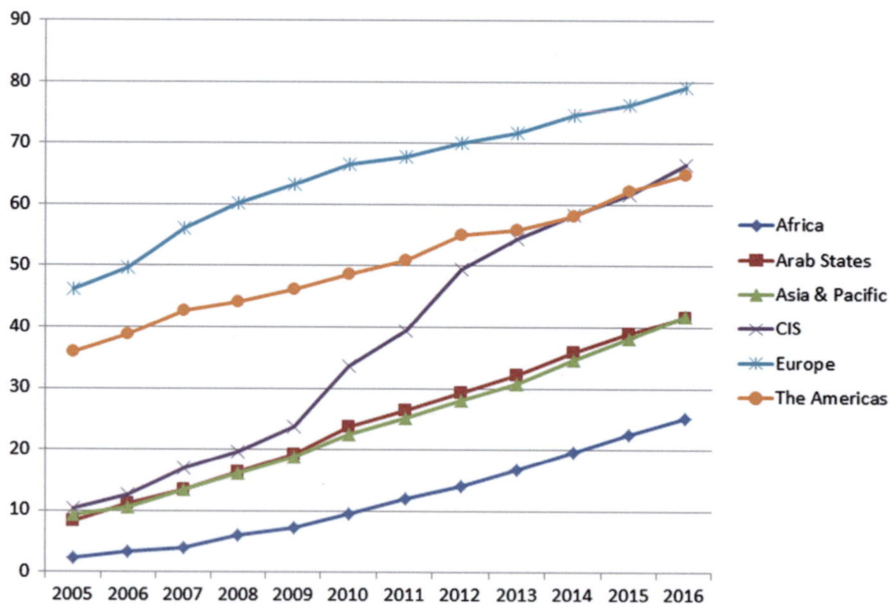

Fig. 13.7 Individuals using the internet (%). My graphics, data from www.itu.int (http://www.itu.int/en/ITU-D/Statistics/Pages/stat/default.aspx)

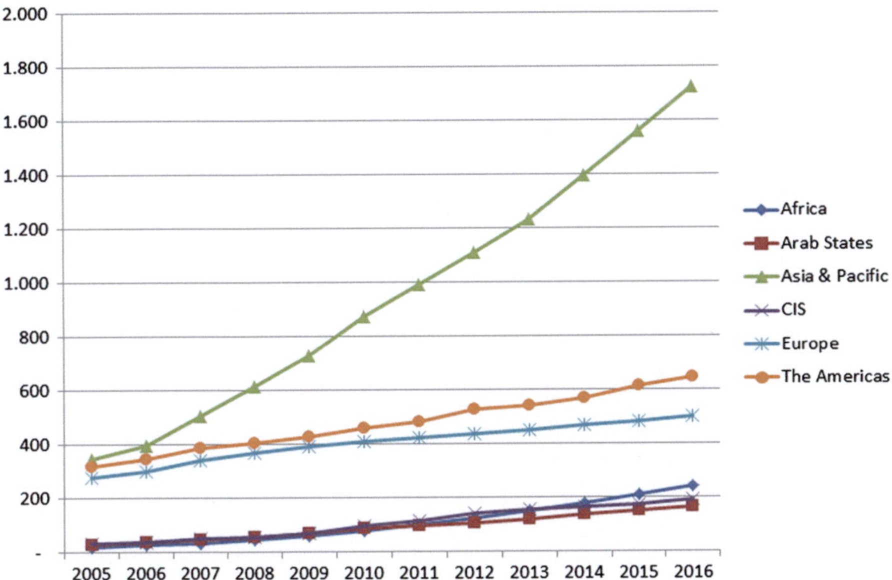

Fig. 13.8 Individuals using the internet (millions). My graphics, data from www.itu.int (http://www.itu.int/en/ITU-D/Statistics/Pages/stat/default.aspx)

References

1. Miller V. Understanding digital culture, 100; 2011.
2. Cole J. I. The UCLA internet report, Surveying the digital future, 5; 2000 (http://www.digitalcenter.org/wp-content/uploads/2012/12/2000_digital_future_report_year1.pdf)
3. Song S. manypossibilities.net
4. http://www.internetworldstats.com/stats.htm

Plant for Africa and Renewable Energy

14

Energy for Life: Electrical Wiring and Renewable Energy Plant Design for Small-Scale Health Facilities in Africa

Giorgio Barbaglia

14.1 Introduction

Mini-grid, micro-grid, smart grid, and renewable energy are the mantras of this last decade in the energy sector [1–3]. These types of hybridization of the traditional electrical grid are a real chance for the future, together with a wider energy mix.

Focusing on Africa, these advances offer an opportunity for emerging countries, giving a chance for development without incurring the past (and present) errors of the "developed" countries.

Many African countries face big problems in many sectors, and essential services such as health, education, clean water, electricity, and transport are not always available. However, Africa also has great potential, not only from the land and sea but also from the African people. It is a young continent, eager for knowledge and new opportunities, and full of good "human energy." Good access to electricity is a basic factor for release of all this human energy. The population increase and urbanization have exponentially increased the demand for power in almost all African countries.

Fifteen years ago, when we started the DREAM program in Mozambique, we had our first face-to-face meeting with African power problems. I still remember the first total blackout of my life in Nampula (Mozambique) in 2003. It was early in the night in the city center, and from my window I could see only the stars and some small red lights moving along the street. I soon discovered that the red lights were just people with lit cigarettes. At that time, we thought that the situation would improve in 10 years at the most. In fact, it did. The availability of electricity in Mozambique has improved in the last decade, but what is the situation in other countries?

The situation seems jeopardized. Focusing on sub-Saharan Africa, the electrification ratio and its growth rate are very different from country to country. We give

G. Barbaglia (✉)
'DREAM Program', Community of Sant'Egidio, Rome, Italy
e-mail: barbigio@gmail.com

© Springer International Publishing AG, part of Springer Nature 2018
M. Bartolo, F. Ferrari (eds.), *Multidisciplinary Teleconsultation in Developing Countries*, TELe-Health, https://doi.org/10.1007/978-3-319-72763-9_14

some examples from countries where DREAM is present and from a "customer" point of view.

Mozambique benefits from the big dam of Cahora Bassa, and invested in the grid so that many rural areas could be reached. Thus, in urban and peri-urban areas, the quality and quantity of electric power has improved dramatically. We should remember that Mozambique was coming out of a very long period of war and the country's infrastructures had to recover from a very bad situation.

Tanzania remains a question mark. It seems that investments are ongoing in the energy sector, but in the summer of 2016, in the north of the country, we experienced a sudden increase in the number and duration of blackouts because of a drop in power production of 35% in one month. The lack of rain caused a crisis in the majority of hydropower plants.

The Republic of Guinea made a large investment in a hydropower plant in Kaletra, which has improved the amount of available power since 2016, mostly reserved for the capital city, Conakry. Less improvement was made in the interior areas. However, the capacity of the dam is not sufficient to keep the turbines 100% active all year. An ancillary dam is necessary to cover power needs during the dry season. The number and duration of blackouts increases as the dry season progresses.

In the Democratic Republic of Congo, the availability of power depends on where you live. The power situation is not so bad in Kinshasa, if you live near the business center of town or near a big hospital or the airport. If you live in the "wrong" place, power and water are not supplied. It is similar in the inner part of the country. In Mbandaka, the capital city of the Equateur Province (more than 400,000 km^2, bigger than Germany), electricity is supplied for some hours in the evening and only in a small part of the town.

How can the situation be improved? In what direction is Africa looking? The increased energy demand is pushing governments to improve power production and distribution. Are mini-grids, micro-grids, or renewable energy on the political agendas and in strategic plans across the continent? Honestly, not so much or not everywhere. Traditional ways of producing and distributing electricity are preferred or seen as most suitable for supporting development; why is this?

There are probably many reasons; however, from an African viewpoint, it seems like a second-best option, an "option B." As happened in other sectors (e.g., the health sector), the "developed world" has planned and proposed options to Africa that are different and without the same appeal as those ("option A") planned and implemented in the developed world. So what looks "cool" to our eyes (renewable energy, micro-grid), what seems to be the future to us, is not considered in the same way in Africa. Big power plants (hydro or thermal with fossil fuels or nuclear) still have a big appeal and the "perfume" of progress.

In Africa, it is not so uncommon to hear someone say "Solar power won't bring development in Africa, it is just a way to impose and sell your technology here." This sounds like they are saying:

You (the developed world) have polluted the world and destroyed a lot of natural resources to support your development, and now you do not want us to reach your level. You want us to remain with limited access to electricity. Solar power or renewable sources will not bring us to your level of prosperity. It is very easy for those who are already 'developed' to talk about a different development model.

Africa is not different from the rest of the world. Every day raises the alarm for global irreversible climate change, a dangerous rise in temperature, and an important loss of rainforest. However, who feels the tragedy of the situation? Who is seriously looking at renewable energy and distributed generation as long-term solutions in the energy sector? We are becoming dangerously accustomed to these alarms; we are getting used to a spoiled planet, to the poverty of the majority, and to the several ongoing wars.

African development can be definitely supported by clean power generation, and Africa can become a model for a different development. However, significant cultural work has to be done in this continent, as in the rest of the world [4].

A "power revolution" can start from where power is still a chimera, but we need a new vision. As long as "development" remains merely equal to "more richness," no new or more sustainable styles of life are possible. If we really love our planet and the complex humanity living on it, deep cultural changes are needed, along with technological innovation in the field of renewable sources.

This is as much a challenge in every continent as it is in Africa.

14.2 Energy for Life

For DREAM, keeping a high standard of health treatment in ten African countries has meant, from the very beginning, facing the problem of an absent or unstable power grid supply.

Treating people effectively is very difficult, sometimes almost impossible, without a reliable source of power. Treatment of HIV patients is a good example. Without good diagnostics, treatments are less effective and definitely risk costing more. Monitoring of key parameters helps reduce the mortality rate among patients on antiretroviral therapy. Effective monitoring reduces treatment failures and results in very low transfer from first- to second-line treatment, which is much more expensive. Use of information technologies (IT) can increase the retention rate and speed up the daily work of health centers and diagnostic laboratories. Telemedicine breaks the barrier and potentially brings a high level of diagnostics everywhere in the world.

The problems were, and still are, the following: running a molecular biology laboratory with $-80\,^{\circ}\mathrm{C}$ ultrafreezer, CD4 count machines, and viral load determination equipment in spite of very frequent and long-lasting blackouts; running an IT infrastructure with the constant risk of losing all data through lack of power; and design a telemedicine service without a reliable source of power.

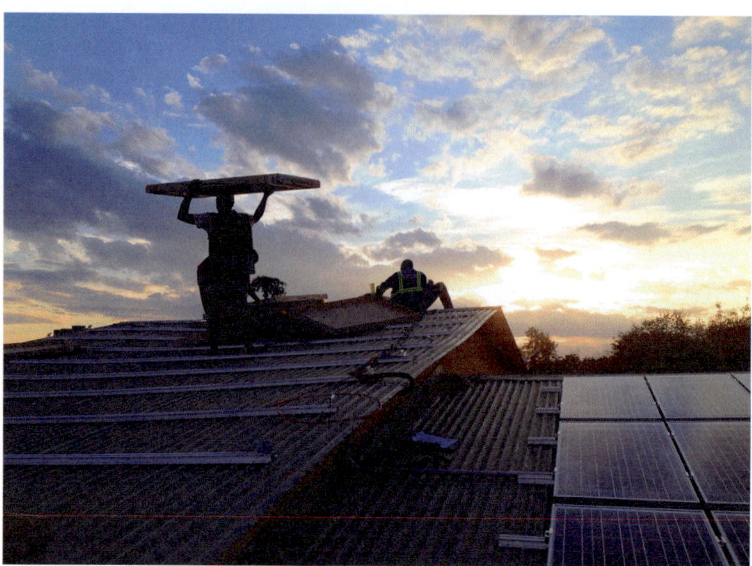

Fig. 14.1 Installing photovoltaic panels on a DREAM center. Balaka, Malawi

From the very beginning, in 2002, we had the idea of using some sort of solar plant to power DREAM health centers and laboratories. However, the very limited budget and the high costs of a solar plant prevented this dream from being realized at that time (Fig. 14.1).

The power situation in sub-Saharan Africa is very different from country to country and from area to area; it is very reliable in some places and absolutely unreliable in others. For DREAM, it was not possible to rely only on the national power grid, which is too volatile, weak, and unstable, with daily and long-lasting blackouts. Moreover, blackouts are usually unpredictable; nobody can advise you that the grid will be off at a specific time. In some countries, where the electricity demand is constantly higher than production capacity, blackouts have a sort of schedule, called load-shedding. This is the case in Malawi, for example. The final result is the same; there is no power for half a day or even more, but you are advised that it can happen. This is a "polite" blackout strategy.

So, we were forced to install a power backup system from the beginning. Installation of a diesel generator set (genset) was a necessity.

14.2.1 Genset

In general, we can consider four ratings in genset operating regimes:

Emergency standby power (ESP)
Limited time running power (LTP)

Table 14.1 Fuel comsumption for diesel generators in DREAM settings

Power generation (kVA)	18	48	110
Diesel consumption (L/h)	3–4	5–6	8–9

Prime running power (PRP)
Continuous operating power (COP)

According to the standard ISO 8528-1:2005, "PRP is the maximum power that a generating set is capable of delivering continuously while supplying a variable electrical load when operated for an unlimited number of hours per year." In addition, when you use a genset at the first two ratings (ESP or LPT), the average power output of the genset should be below 70% of the PRP. It is also true that, for ESP or LTP, an oversized genset consumes less and lasts longer. However, it is recommended not to oversize too much to avoid moving too far from the best efficiency point of the engine (normally close to 75% of the maximum load). In the case of DREAM, diesel gensets have been installed with powers ranging from 18 to 110 kVA, depending on the load profile of the facility to be powered.

Fuel consumption of a diesel genset (like that of a car or truck) depends on several factors, the main ones being engine design, load, age, and maintenance. Table 14.1 lists some average values from DREAM field experience, recorded over long periods (years) for the LTP case. They may be slightly different from values declared by the manufacturers.

To operate the genset and to switch between the main source of power (grid) and the backup source (genset), either a manual or automatic transfer switch can be used. In DREAM facilities, the need for freezers to be kept at $-80\,^{\circ}\text{C}$ (a nightmare for the technical service), overnight critical laboratory analysis, and data servers on 24 h forced us to have a reliable system that can power crucial equipment day and night without any interruption. Therefore, installation of an automatic transfer switch (ATS) was mandatory.

It is obvious that if a power grid is available and the genset is only used as a backup system, the running costs remain within reasonable limits. However, if the number of blackouts increases and their durations become hours or days, genset operation approaches the COP rating, meaning that fuel and maintenance costs become very important.

We should also consider that each blackout means that the genset starts and the ATS switches from the main source to the backup and then back when the main source becomes available again. Thus, a large number of blackouts causes mechanical stress for the cranking of the engine, the battery on board the genset, and the ATS. In Conakry, we measured up to 25 blackouts in a single day (25 start/stops of the genset, 50 toggles of the ATS). Long-duration blackouts also mean that maintenance (oil, filters, etc.) of the genset is needed more frequently. In hot and dusty locations, manufacturers recommend maintenance every 250 operating hours. However, in Conakry, Mthengo wa Ntenga (Malawi), and Usa River (Tanzania), we were sometimes close to 300 genset hours per month and were forced to service the genset every month. Genset maintenance costs should also be seriously considered.

With a backup genset, you feel safe, but what about failure of the genset? Furthermore, what happens if the failure is something serious or occurs during a long-lasting blackout or load-shedding? This is a real problem. Mechanics are not normally available quickly on site, and sometimes spare parts are out of stock in the country and have to be ordered overseas. If the equipment is protected by an uninterruptible power supply (UPS) (see Sect. 14.2.2), there is time to stop some services and shut down the computers and the servers, but what about the $-80\,^\circ$C ultrafreezers or long incubation analyses? What about the daily routine? Is it possible to stop all IT services or laboratory analyses at any blackout and simply start them again when the grid is functioning again? In such a critical situation, a second small backup genset can be useful. It does not need to be very big, just the correct size to power all the critical loads or at least the central UPS (see Sect. 14.2.2). This also means that a second transfer switch should be installed from genset1 to genset2.

A diesel genset is not the only essential item. A genset alone does not prevent all computers, servers, or laboratory machines from turning off in the case of a blackout or micro-interruption in the power supply. A UPS is another must-have in DREAM facilities.

14.2.2 Uninterruptible Power Supply

What kind of UPS is most appropriate and what size? How big does the battery pack need to be?

Where the need is only to protect some computers and other small pieces of equipment, a traditional small UPS is the right choice. These typically range between 500 and 1000 W with 10 min of battery runtime. For a complete molecular laboratory equipped with a $-80\,^\circ$C ultrafreezer and other high power consuming machines, the installation of a central three-phase UPS is mandatory. How big does this UPS need to be?

The decision process is very similar to that for choosing the correct genset. In this case, it is true that an oversized UPS will last longer. A good rule is to find the best compromise between the requirement and the money available. A good base point is not to exceed 70% of the UPS maximum power. If possible, the load should stay under 50-60% of the UPS maximum power (in this case, a future increase in load can be accommodated). A central UPS (a good choice is the online double conversion type) can be quite expensive, so it is very important to analyze which loads are critical and should be protected by the UPS and which are not. It is not necessary to power everything through the UPS. Heating devices such as water distillers, sterilizers, and air conditioning (AC) systems may not need to be on the UPS output line. Much of the lighting system could also be excluded.

If a plumber or other specialist has to do some work in the health center, it is important that the soldering machine or other equipment is not pugged into the UPS output!! For this reason, it is better that the UPS sockets are different from normal sockets and that normal plugs cannot fit inside a UPS socket. Personnel should be instructed and advised on how to use the different kinds of sockets; but, it can happen that a new person joins the staff or someone not part of the staff has some work to do (remember the plumber and the soldering machine).

Separating what is critical and what is not requires installation of at least two separate distribution boards (DB), one on the UPS output, powering all critical loads, and the other on the national power grid line, powering all items that can stay off until the genset is functioning. The exercise of minimizing the load will be very useful when considering solar plants.

How big should the UPS battery pack be? To answer this, we should anticipate some issues that will be encountered again when talking about solar batteries.

Batteries are a big family (and the family is growing every day) with very different features for each of the members. For the moment, we will focus on the lead-acid batteries that are still the most popular technology for UPS units, mainly because of their lower cost, simple connection to the DC busbar, electrical safety, and reliability. In particular, we consider sealed batteries that do not need maintenance.

This kind of battery does not have a very long life and is also very delicate. They should not be discharged too much below the declared depth of discharge (DOD) and they cannot be cycled (charged/discharged) indefinitely. Depending on the manufacturing technology, the lifecycle ranges from some hundreds of cycles to a maximum of 2000–2500 cycles, but not with deep discharge. Inside a three-phase UPS, the voltage across the battery pack is normally close to 400 V. This means that a large number of batteries in series are needed, because the typical nominal voltage on a UPS lead-acid battery is 12 V. When you start having problems with some batteries of the pack, it is wise to replace the whole pack. It is not a good idea to have new batteries together with old and exploited batteries in the same array. This means that, normally, at least 32 batteries need replacing at the same time, a factor to be considered in calculating the budget.

Coming back to the question of the size of the UPS, if the budget allows, a large number of batteries can assure a very long and conformable runtime. However, they will need replacing after some years, which will affect the running costs budget. Therefore, this item should be sized not only on the basis of technical requirements and the operational needs of the moment, but also with an eye on the future budget.

14.2.3 Voltage Regulator and More

Blackouts are not the only problem related to use of the power grid. A central UPS normally has a log function, which we have used to record many problems from the grid over the last 15 years. We have noted overvoltages and undervoltages, sometimes very far from the rated value of 400 V three phase or 230 V single phase (in some places you can still find 380 V three phase and 220 V single phase); surges, spikes, strange variations in frequency to over or even under the rated value of 50 Hz, phase drops and, worst of all, neutral drops. It is a daily battle and it is impossible to stay protected from every strange occurrence. However, at the very beginning we decided to install a voltage regulator just after the grid meter. We chose a traditional electromechanical type with three independent coils and regulators. This was a good choice for the strength of the machine and its easy maintenance.

In addition, when building a health facility plus a laboratory with installed power of over 20–30 kVA, be prepared to install your own medium voltage (MV) powerhouse, or at least a pole transformer with protection devices. Often, when you ask the national provider for anything over 20 kVA, they answer that the local transformer is too small or already full, so the only possibility is a MV three-phase connection. This happened to us almost everywhere we installed a laboratory.

We can summarize a typical DREAM electrical installation as including the following elements:

- MV powerhouse or MV pole transformer (130–150 kVA)
- Three-phase meter (unfortunately, we need to pay for the electricity we use!)
- Three-phase surge protector system (storms and lightening are frequent and dangerous in tropical and equatorial regions)
- Three-phase voltage regulator (110 kVA)
- One main DB
- One ATS (three phase, 120 A)
- One or two gensets (the big one around 100 kVA, the small one around 40 kVA)
- One sub-DB from the grid to power noncritical loads. The more the loads can be divided into separate lines, the better operational continuity can be assured. Thus, a problem with one piece of equipment that causes a miniature circuit breaker (MCB) or residual current circuit breaker (RCCB) to trip affects only a limited sector of the building.
- One central three-phase UPS (40 kVA with 30 min run time battery pack)
- One sub-DB from the UPS to power critical loads. Without overcomplicating the DBs, the points mentioned for noncritical sub-DBs are also valid here.

14.3 The Solar Dream

Sub-Saharan African power grids are improving, but there is still a long way to go. To become self-sufficient and produce your own power is an attractive solution. Producing power in a clean way also means taking care the future of our planet. Helping neighbors with your surplus of clean power improves solidarity and community links.

DREAM obtained the opportunity to use a renewable source of power in 2012, when we received a specific grant to upgrade our electrical installations with the use of solar power in Malawi. Malawi is a small and beautiful country that is very important in the DREAM network. Several DREAM health centers and three complete laboratories cover the central and south part of the country. The national power situation has all the problems already explained, so it was very good news that our solar dream might come true. Once the renewable source (the sun) was chosen, many questions emerged in our discussions: What size should the solar plant be? Should the system be off-grid, on-grid, or hybrid? How many and what type of PV

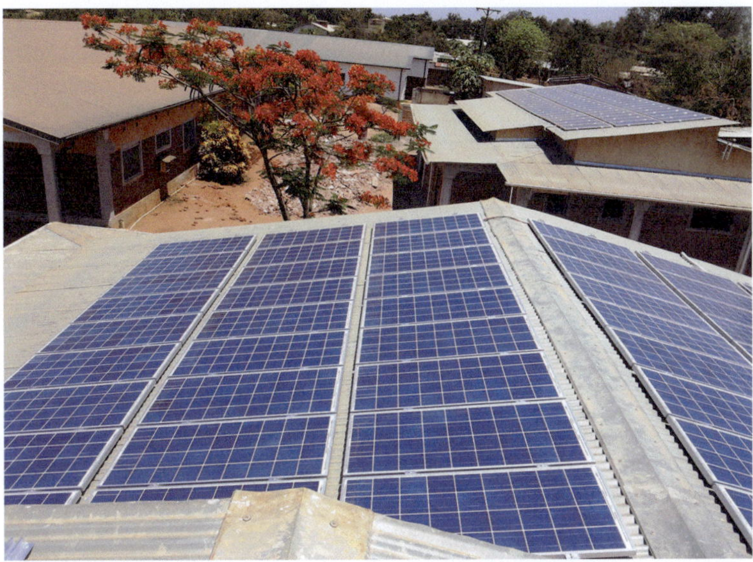

Fig. 14.2 Solar plant on DREAM center. Balaka, Malawi

panels should be installed? Which technology and brand for the inverter and solar charger should be chosen? What type of storage should be used and how big? What type of battery is most appropriate? Should the PV panels be on the roof or on the ground? Furthermore, we were dealing with already existing and operational facilities, with proper and complex power systems and wirings. The starting point was not a blank page (Fig. 14.2).

14.4   The Sizing Process

We have three types of facilities: (i) large health center + complete diagnostics laboratory + telemedicine, (ii) health center + telemedicine, and (iii) small health center.

Focusing first on the large health center, it was immediately clear that it would not be financially viable to use a solar plant to power all the loads. A single solar plant would drain the budget. Fortunately, the wiring was already well done, with specific power lines to each room of the laboratory, the computer network, server room, different sectors of the lighting system, and the different AC units. It was therefore easy to move the different loads in and out and finally put the puzzle together.

What was already on the central UPS output was automatically included in the solar-powered system, plus lights and some of the drug store and laboratory ACs (laboratory temperature should remain within a stable range; otherwise, some diagnostic equipment can become out of calibration and refuse to start).

As a rough calculation, assuming all loads in the solar basket are on at the same time, the sum of their power loads gives the maximum power (in kilowatts) needed from the solar inverter. To calculate the energy (in kilowatt hours) needed in a day or week, we need to know for how long each piece of equipment is used in a day or, better, in a week (assuming that all routine operations are included in a week). However, when dealing with solar power and solar batteries, it is better to be accurate. The best way to avoid errors is to install a network analyzer (or at least an energy meter) on the input line of the solar power DB (in this phase of the project, it is still the DB of the UPS). With an accurate load profile, or at least with an average weekly energy demand, we can calculate the PV panels and solar batteries needed. For an off-grid system, it is very important to have separate day/night load profiles to determine the size of battery storage required. We soon discovered the advantages and disadvantages of each configuration, as summarized below [5]:

Off-grid system
- Pros: Completely autonomous, no grid problems, zero energy bill
- Cons: Higher initial cost (more panels and more batteries needed), higher maintenance cost (when changing the battery pack)

On-grid system
- Its canonical implementation (with the metering option) was impossible. The Malawi power grid was not designed to receive our surplus solar production. The situation is the same in other African countries.

Hybrid system (PV panels, battery storage, power grid, diesel genset)
- Pros: Lower initial cost (battery pack can be smaller and, in our case, a diesel genset was already present), lower maintenance cost (when changing the battery pack).
- Cons: Higher technical complexity and the need for supervisory control (a data acquisition system is advantageous in helping tune up the plant); severe grid problems could still affect the system, and genset problems are still possible.

In 2012, solar hybrid power systems were still in the first stage of commercialization for private consumers. Nobody had any relevant experience with them. However, this option sounded good to us because we already had the grid and the genset to power the DREAM installations, which lowered the cost considerably compared with an off-grid solution. The extra cost of the more complex electronics seemed much smaller than the extra cost of the battery pack needed for the off-grid solution. Finally, we took the risk and fortunately found a good manufacturer/supplier. After some inquiries in Malawi and in Europe, we decided to buy all the materials in Europe; the total cost (including shipping and fees) was dramatically lower than in Malawi (the other reason was that not everything was available in the country). This is another point to consider; the solar market in many African countries is not mature and the prices are still very high.

14.4.1 Hybrid Solar–Grid–Diesel DREAM Plant

We finally chose an Italian product, Sirio Power Supply (SPS) [6], manufactured by AROS Solar. Two of the advantages of this system were the reasonable price and the

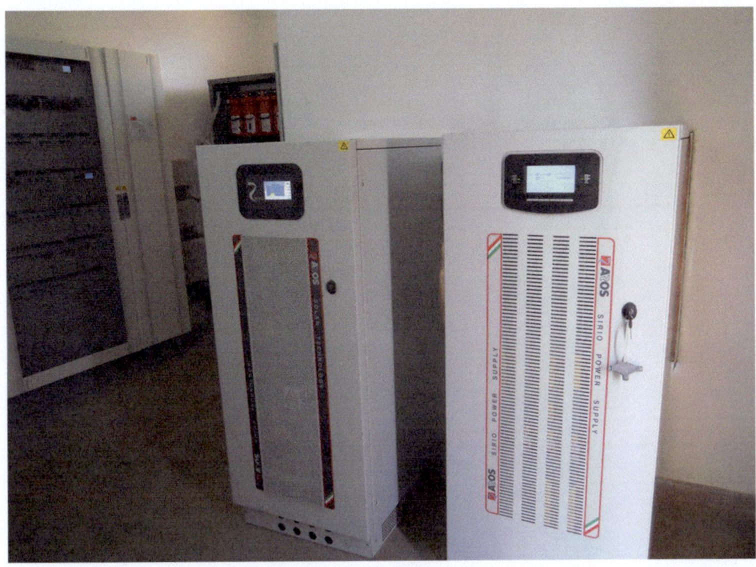

Fig. 14.3 AROS SPS hybrid solar inverters powering DREAM center and laboratory. Balaka, Malawi

very friendly assistance we received. Their engineers agreed to study our case and adapt their products to our specific situation.

Figures 14.3, 14.4, 14.5, 14.6, 14.7 show the layout and the different operating conditions of the three solar plants installed in Malawi in 2013 and 2014 and in the Republic of Guinea in 2015.

Condition 1: With sufficient sunlight, the PV inverter powers the load and charges the battery through the bidirectional SPS output; grid and genset are off.

Condition 2: With insufficient sunlight, the load is powered by the PV inverter with the aid of the battery. For optimum use of the genset, the battery discharge level can be set.

Condition 3a: With lack of sunlight, the PV inverter is off or does not produce enough power. Here, the battery has reached 10% of the DOD and the grid is present. The load is completely/partially supplied by the grid, and the grid also recharges the battery.

Condition 3b: With lack of sunlight, the PV inverter is off or does not produce enough power. Here, the battery has reached 30% of the DOD and the grid is not present. The load is completely/partially supplied by the genset, and the genset also recharges the battery.

- In conditions 1, 2, and 3a, if sunlight is present/returns and is sufficient to power the load, the PV inverter overrides any current operation.
- In condition 3b, even when sunlight returns, the genset remains on until the battery has reach at least 90% charge.

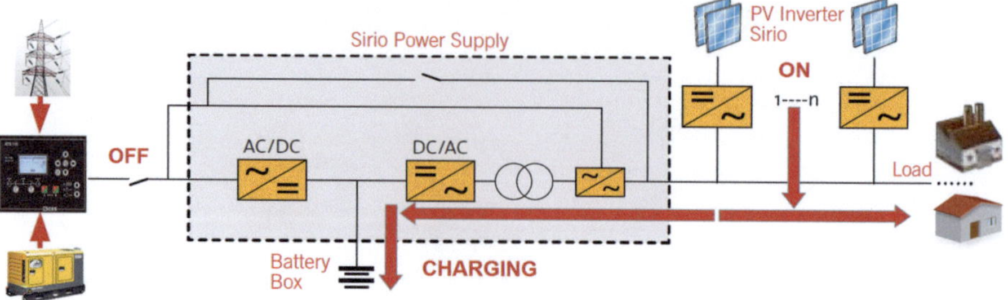

Fig. 14.4 Condition 1 (courtesy of Aros-Solar)

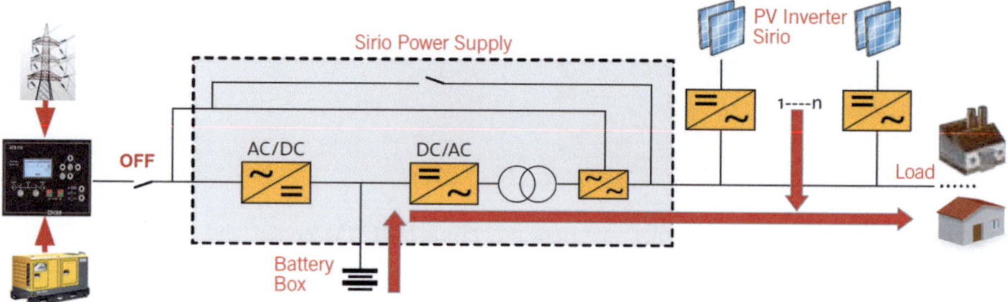

Fig. 14.5 Condition 2 (courtesy of Aros-Solar)

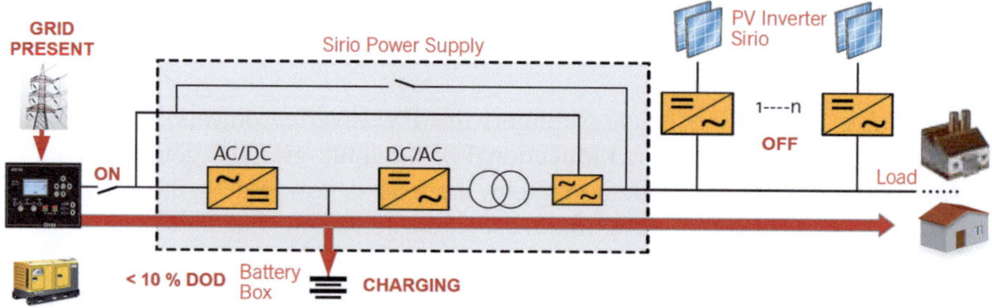

Fig. 14.6 Condition 3a (courtesy of Aros-Solar)

- In the worst condition (no sunlight, no grid, and genset failure), the system discharges the battery until 50% of DOD, then drops the load to preserve battery life.
- The supervisory logic on board the SPS controls all parameters and also the start and stop of the genset.
- All parameters are adjustable from the control panel of the SPS.
- The two values of 10% and 30% for the DOD of the battery are very conservative values and come from our field experience.

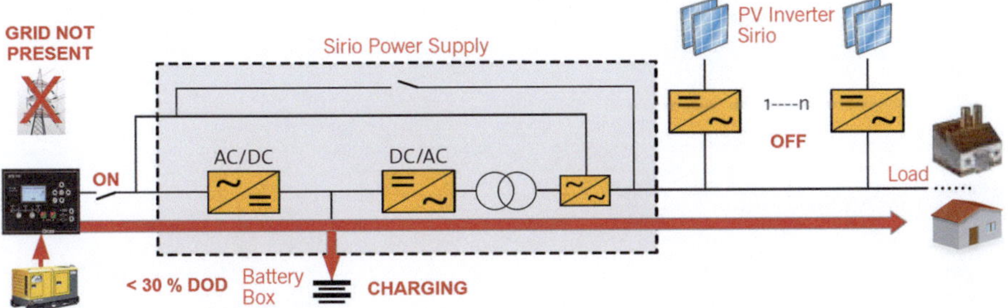

Fig. 14.7 Condition 3b (courtesy of Aros-Solar)

The layout was finally clear, but many questions remained: What type of PV panels should be used? How many kilowatts peak (kWp) of solar production are needed? Where should we install the panels? How many batteries are needed? What type of battery should we choose? Where should we install the batteries? Where should we install the SPS?

Our conclusions were made after many discussions, consultations with experts (I should say they were more "friends" than "consultants"), and market surveys.

14.4.2 Photovoltaic Panels [7]

Using a high DC voltage maximum power point tracking (MPPT) [8] inverter, almost any kind of PV panel can be used. The temperature sensitivity of the panel can be used as a parameter to discriminate between one or the other. However, the cost of PV panels has dropped considerably in the last decade, so it is better to install as many panels as possible. If the average load is 20 kW, it is better to install 30 or 35 kWp of solar panels.

A large number of panels can keep solar production high, even in sub-optimal sunlight situations, which prevents the battery pack from discharging. A high DC voltage MPPT inverter allows a series of about 20 panels (string of panels), producing a high DC voltage (over 600 V) that allows low currents and consequently small sized wires (Fig. 14.8).

Installing the panels on the ground is more expensive than on a roof (you need the support to be firmly grounded) and needs an adequate piece of land. In addition, the panels must be protected with a fence to prevent someone from damaging or stealing them, and also for safety reasons because of the high DC voltage. However, cleaning and maintenance are much easier. Installation on an existing roof is quicker and cheaper, but raises the problem of panel ventilation to prevent their temperature from increasing too much (PV panel efficiency decreases with increasing temperature). Future maintenance or cleaning operations are more difficult, but a fence is not needed and it is more difficult for someone to damage or steal the panels.

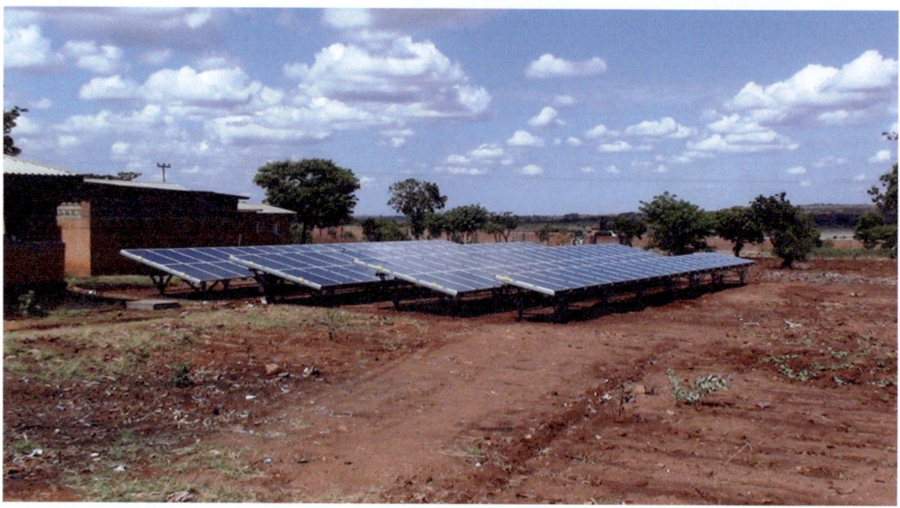

Fig. 14.8 Photovoltaic solar plant powering DREAM center and laboratory. Mthengo wa Ntenga (Lilongwe) Malawi

It is important to avoid any shadow on the panels, which dramatically decreases the efficiency of the string. Keep the panels as clean as possible, particularly in dusty places and during long dry seasons. Cut the grass if panels are on the ground!

Tilt and orientation were initially a big concern, but we discovered that if you are not far from the equator, they have a very slightly impact on solar production. It is better to install some extra panels and not worry too much about tilt and orientation. However, altitude and level of humidity in the air have a remarkable impact on the efficiency of the panels. The same PV panel installed in Malawi in a dry area at 1150 m above sea level was 15–20% more efficient than in Conakry, with wet atmosphere at sea level.

14.4.3 Batteries [9]

Energy storage is an important issue. The most common solution is to use electro-chemical accumulators. As mentioned in the UPS description (Sect. 14.2.2), there are very many types of batteries and continuous research in this field adds new members to the family every year (just consider what is happening in the automotive sector) (Fig. 14.9).

It is quite easy to find lists, descriptions, and ratings of the different types of batteries. Here, we only consider the two extremes in terms of cost. Lead-acid batteries are the cheapest type. They are available in different shapes and as dry, wet, absorbent glass mat (AGM), sealed/unsealed, with/without maintenance, nor-mal/deep cycle, specific for solar/automotive installation or for logistic equipment such as forklifts, valve regulated, gel, OPzS, with straight or tubular elements, flooded, free acid, and many combinations of these types and features. In general,

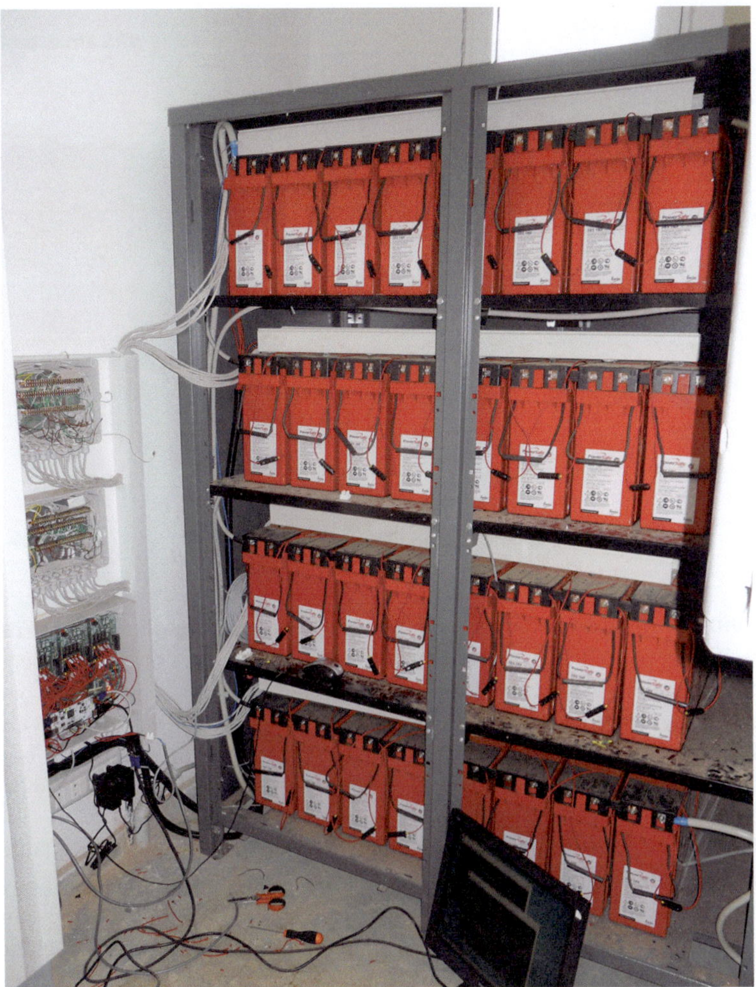

Fig. 14.9 Installing battery packs and monitoring system in the power room side of the DREAM molecular laboratory. Balaka, Malawi

the more you pay, the better performance obtained in terms of capacity, DOD, and duration in years. At present, batteries are the most expensive component of a solar power plant. Thus, the choice of battery is very much dependent on the budget. A specific battery for solar applications can last four times longer than a basic lead-acid battery, but it costs four times more. So, the choice is very much related to the initial budget.

The voltage across the battery should also be considered. Batteries for solar application are traditionally 2 V batteries. In our specific case, the SPS required about 400 V on the battery pack. This strongly limited our choice. To avoid an enormous number of batteries, we were forced to choose 12 V batteries.

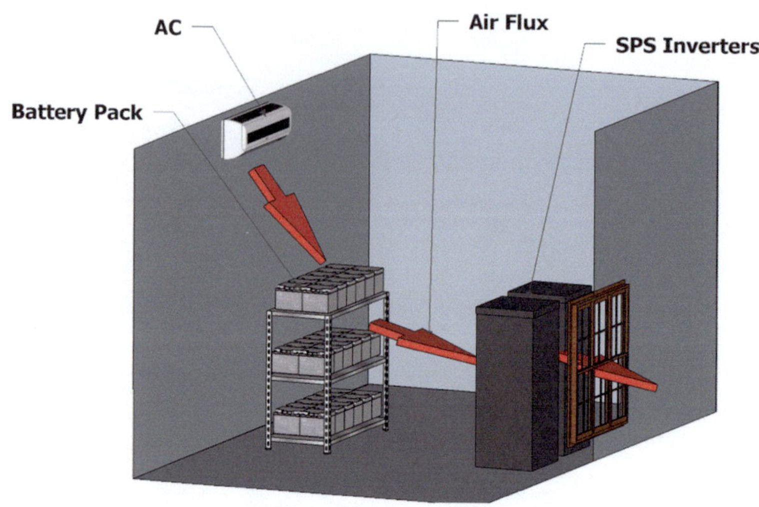

Fig. 14.10 Typical batteries, inverter, air conditioner layout

Lithium-ion (Li-ion) batteries were the most expensive at that time. With DOD close to 100%, an impressive number of cycles, and a very long life, it seems that they are the future, even in solar applications. Many big companies are working on this technology and the market prices are rapidly decreasing; things are changing very fast in the storage sector. Many new integrated products are also becoming available, including a MPPT solar charger, an inverter, an advance battery manager, and a Li-ion battery pack in one box.

DREAM's specific use of the facilities is such that they are operational during the day and closed during the night, with minimal services running. We therefore chose to install a minimal battery pack in order to save money and increase the number of sites where we would be able to install solar power systems. Our choice was 32 AGM lead-acid batteries of 200 Ah with enhanced DOD and life cycle, representing a good compromise between performance and cost. To keep the batteries in good shape for as long as possible, we decided to use them in a very conservative way (10% DOD if grid is present, 30% if not). AGM batteries are also very sensitive to temperature, so the temperature of the battery room needs to be controlled as much as possible. The better the room temperature can be maintained at 25 °C, the longer the batteries will last. A typical DREAM installation is shown in Fig. 14.10.

AC increases the load and power consumption, but tests showed that the extra cost is worth it for a 30 kW solar installation. The negative impact on the power consumption is easily compensated by better battery performance and their longer duration. It is clear that the use of solar production is not maximized, but the highest cost is not the grid power bill in Malawi and in the other African countries where we installed our solar plants. If a good and stable grid is present, there are no economic reasons to install a private solar plant (although environmental protection reasons are always valid). The cost of fuel for the diesel genset is higher. With this kind of hybrid solar installation, we have not reduced use of the genset to zero, but reduced it by a factor of 10. We have not reduced our grid electricity bill to zero, but reduced it by a factor of 3. In Conakry, for example, in 2015 we used the diesel genset for an average of 250 h per month. After installation of the SPS solar plant, we used the genset for an average of 20 h per month. The environment smiles and also our accountants. Note that only essential services are powered by solar energy in DREAM facilities. The rest of the load remains on the grid or on the genset if it is running. This has two important consequences: the electricity bill is not zero and nonessential services are off during blackouts (note, there may be complaints if the AC is off for long time).

As discussed, keeping only essential services under solar power allowed us to minimize the solar power system and tailor it to our needs, saving a lot of money. Remember that, in the majority of African countries, it is not possible to feed any power surplus into the grid.

14.4.4 Small-Size Solar Plants

The solar power system described above was installed in DREAM centers with total installed power of over 40 kW and essential services power of about 20 kW.

In small-sized DREAM facilities (i.e., four to six rooms, no laboratory, and maybe with telemedicine), about 2–3 kW are sufficient to run the computers, lights, and telemedicine service. In this case, an off-grid traditional solar installation can meet the requirements. The problem of having a consistent battery pack remains. If only solar power is used to run the health facility, the number of PV panels and batteries installed should provide sufficient run time, even in bad weather conditions. Only a few DREAM centers are in rural areas not served by the electric grid. So, for small DREAM facilities our choice was also a hybrid solar power system. This allows us to use grid power when present (Fig. 14.11).

Figure 14.12 shows an example of such installations used in Malawi and Tanzania. After a market survey, we found the best compromise between cost and reliability in the Ensolar brand distributed by Entrade [10]. These are small-size hybrid solar inverters. We are using the 2 kW and 3.5 kW models. No genset is installed in this kind of DREAM facility, so the only sources of power are sun, batteries, and grid.

As described for the SPS AROS Solar system, the priorities are as follows:

– PV panels, if solar irradiation is sufficient to power the load and keep the battery pack charged
– PV panels + batteries, if irradiation is not sufficient
– Grid, if no or insufficient irradiation and the batteries are discharging too much

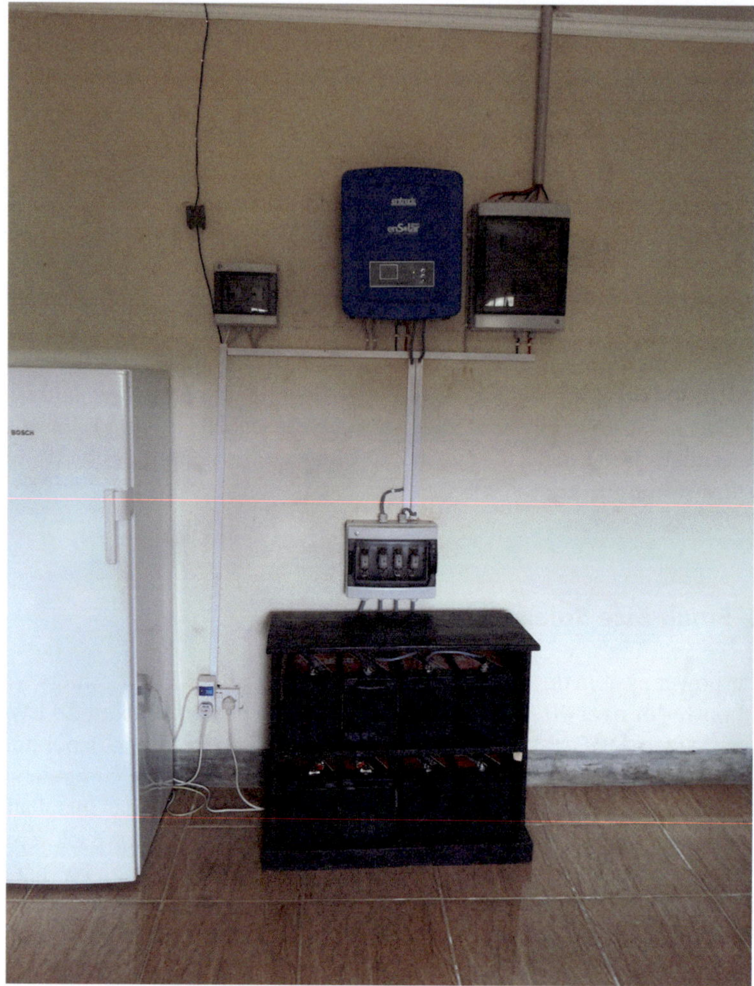

Fig. 14.11 Small-size hybrid solar inverter plus batteries at the DREAM Nutritional Center. Machinjiri (Blantyre) Malawi

In this case, it is not possible to control the DOD of the batteries, so the factory preset is used. The battery packs in these installations are small because a long run time is not needed during the day and no load is connected during the night. It is possible that the worst situation of no sun, discharged batteries, and no grid can occur, but it is not very common. Thus, a small investment in batteries is normally sufficient to supply the daily needs of the DREAM operation.

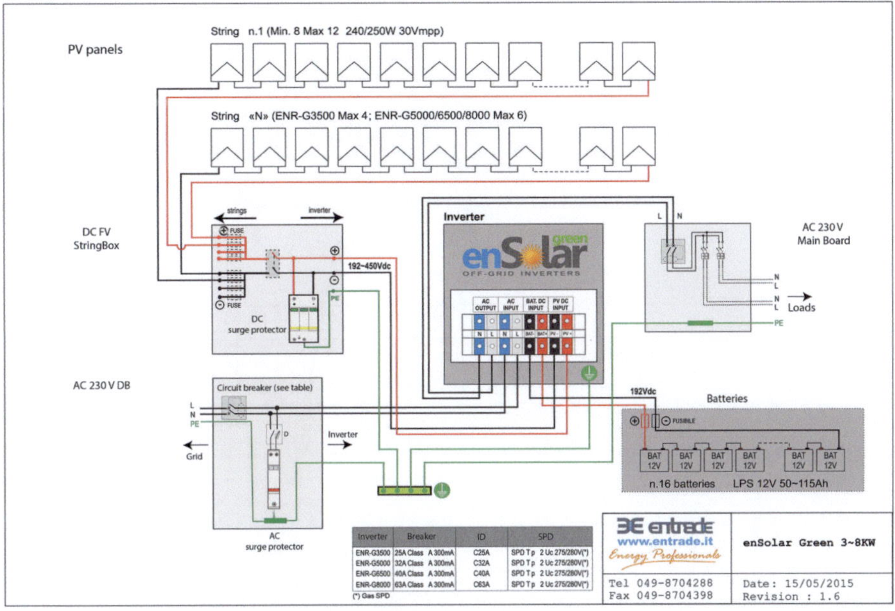

Fig. 14.12 Ensolar 3kW to 6kW typical layout (courtesy of Entrade)

14.4.5 Data Collection

In all our large solar installations, we installed a data logger system and receive daily information from the solar plants, including the following useful parameters:

– PV voltage and current
– Battery pack voltage and current
– Grid voltages and currents
– SPS output voltages and currents
– Voltage and temperature of each battery

All these parameters are logged each minute and sent via the internet (DREAM centers already have an internet connection for other purposes). It is a large amount of data but very important for monitoring the health of the system.

In the beginning, just after commissioning the plant, these data are very useful for tuning the system (equilibration of phases at different moments of the workday, battery pack DOD thresholds). After commissioning, such data are essential to keep the weakest parts of the system in good health; for example, a drop in battery pack voltage or an increase in temperature are bad signs. In the SPS system, all batteries are in series so failure of one battery leads to failure of the whole system and probably to damage of other batteries in the same pack. Prompt information about the incoming problem can avoid this.

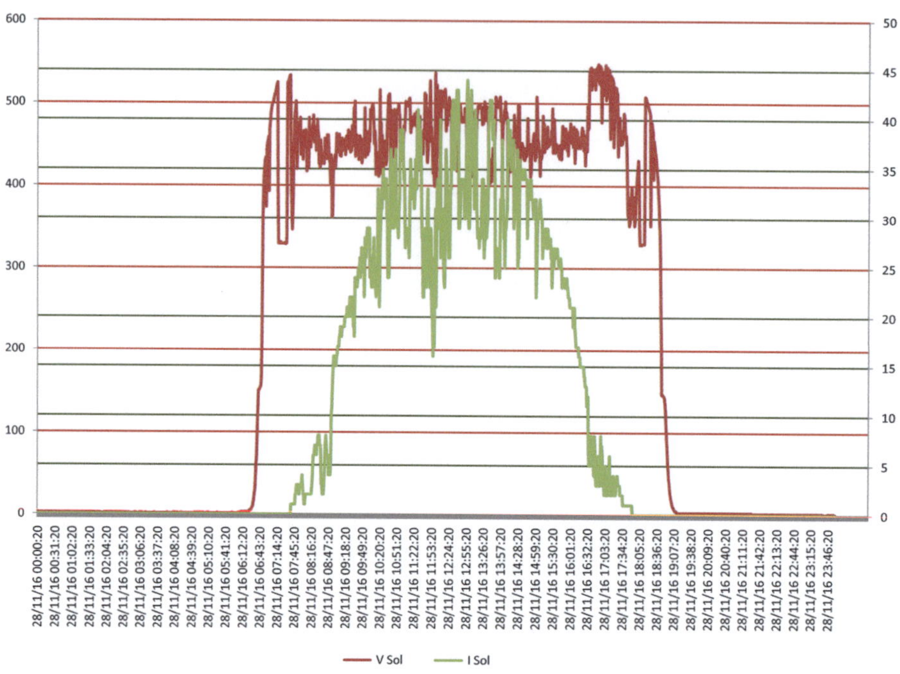

Fig. 14.13 Photovoltaic voltage (V) and current (A) on a 24-h basis

The data logger/monitoring system helps prevent this kind of problem. Through the collected data, we can also know the following:

– PV production evolution during any period of interest
– Grid presence and quality
– Genset usage
– Battery pack usage
– Any statistic or trend analysis required

Some examples of possible graphs are given in Figs. 14.13 and 14.14.

14.5 Environmental Protection and Climate Change

So far, we have focused on the technical feasibility and economic viability of the use of pure solar or hybrid solar power plants to power health facilities in sub-Saharan Africa. We have demonstrated that it is technically possible and economically viable, but beyond any technical or economic aspects, solar power is the way for the future. No sustainable future development can rely on traditional fossil power sources.

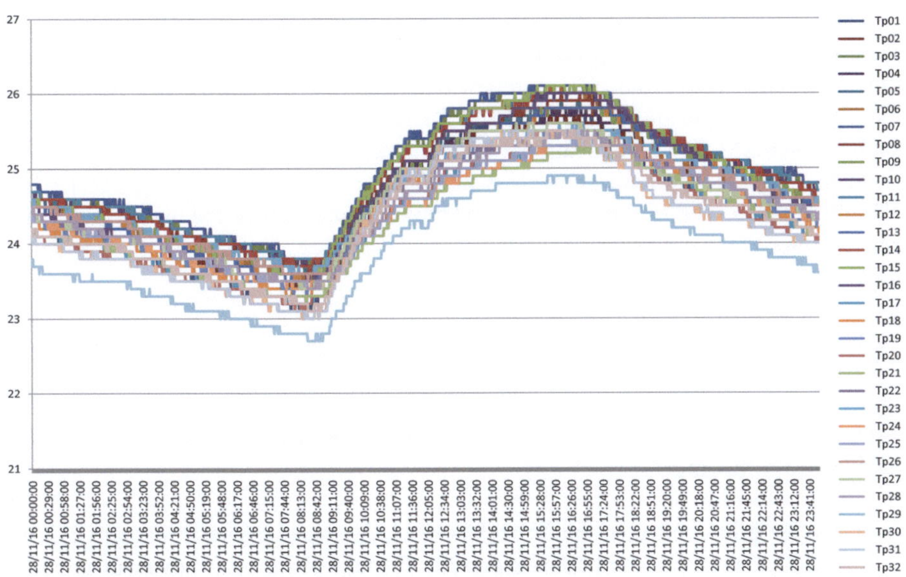

Fig. 14.14 Battery temperature (°C) on a 24-h basis

We will need more electricity (electricity will be the future "fuel" in the automotive sector) and we will need to produce it in a cleaner way. We can try to justify our delay or postpone historic decisions, but "force majeure" will soon force us to change our way of dealing with power generation.

Africa has a big opportunity not to follow the wrong path taken by the so-called developed countries in the last century. Africa has the opportunity to take advantages of the mistakes made by other continents in recent years. Some big African cities are already among the most polluted in the world, so it is time that Africa makes decisions. Climate change has accelerated in recent years and it is not a time to look on silently. Distributed electricity generation from renewable sources can be a chance for many countries, especially in the wide spaces of rural Africa.

For every liter of diesel burnt, 2650 g of CO_2 is released. Replacing a 100 kVA diesel genset with a solar power system or recycling it as part of a hybrid solar power system (as we did) prevents the release of about 40 tons of CO_2 each year. It is difficult to say how many diesel generators are installed in sub-Saharan Africa and how many people are using them for self-production of power. Different sector studies and outlooks indicate that in 2017 the number of diesel generators sold in sub-Saharan Africa will reach 19,000 units, most of which are diesel generators of over 100 kVA. The trend is positive, so more than 20,000 new diesel generators will be installed each year from now on; this means millions of tons of CO_2 released into the atmosphere each year.

From our experience, we think that health centers such as the DREAM program facilities, are good starting point for the development of a micro/mini-grid in Africa. Often, sceptics about the use of renewable energies emphasize the problem of management of distributed generation of energy; why not start with health centers such as DREAM or with educational institutions?

In these cases, the management, maintenance system, and security service are already in place. The health center can be the first customer of the micro-grid and it can become the focal point of other kinds of services, like electricity, through a micro-grid.

14.6 Conclusions

After 4 years of solar energy usage in the DREAM program across Africa, we have learned the following:

- If you are grid-connected, but use a 80–100 kVA diesel genset as backup unit for 150–200 h a month, the payback period of your hybrid solar power installation can easily be very close to 4 years. This is much shorter than for a typical on-grid installation.
- A hybrid solar power installation is a very low maintenance system. All that is required is to keep the panels clean and keep the batteries as fresh as possible.
- With a hybrid solar power system, any reasonable increase in load is possible and will not constrain future expansion of telemedicine or laboratory equipment. In our design for the hybrid power system, batteries act as a "flywheel" and not as real storage. It is not necessary to change or improve the battery pack if the load is increased (to improve a battery pack after some time is hard, but to add fresh batteries to an old battery pack is not recommended). Thus, the only limits are the inverter power and the PV field installed power.
- A hybrid solar power system reduces the stress in cases of long grid failure (sometimes 3 or 4 days without electricity), making management of the genset easier. Less time on genset means less fuel to buy or stock, less genset maintenance, and less panic and calls for technical assistance if the engine does not start when needed.
- A side effect of solar power installation is an improvement in the skills of local engineers and technicians. Through African and European technicians working together on sizing of the hybrid solar system and its installation, the competence of technicians involved has improved. These are skills very useful for DREAM in maintaining the installed solar plants, but are also skills that technicians can use everywhere in their daily work (Fig. 14.15).
- Another desirable side effect for the near future is to have surplus power that can be used to help neighbors and improve the interaction between the health center and the surround community.
- A primary outcome of the solar power installations is tons of CO_2 less in the African sky, giving a smaller carbon footprint.

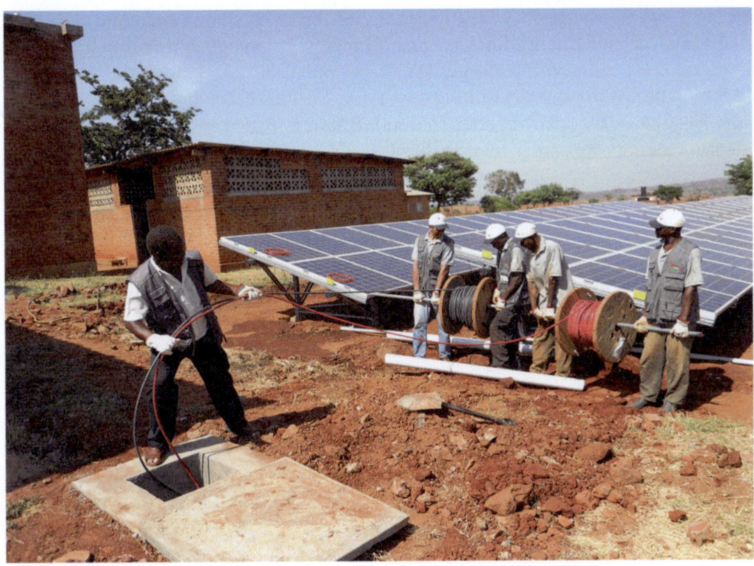

Fig. 14.15 Installing a hybrid solar power system at the DREAM center and laboratory. Mthengo wa Ntenga (Lilongwe) Malawi

The DREAM solar installations are positive, visible, and durable examples showing that it is possible to provide good health services with a smaller impact on the planet.

References

1. Kim HM, Kinoshita T. A new challenge of microgrid operation. In: Kim T, Stoica A, Chang RS, editors. Security-enriched urban computing and smart grid. Communications in computer and information science, vol. 78. Berlin, Heidelberg: Springer; 2010.
2. Farimani FD, Mashhadi HR. Modeling and implementation of demand dispatch approach in a smart micro-grid. In: Constanda C, Kirsch A, editors. Integral methods in science and engineering. Cham: Birkhäuser; 2015.
3. Mithulananthan N, Hung DQ, Lee KY. Intelligent network integration of distributed renewable generation. Cham: Springer; 2017.
4. Bhattacharyya SC, Palit D. Mini-grids for rural electrification of developing countries. Cham: Springer; 2014.
5. Karthikeyan V, Rajasekar S, Das V, Karuppanan P, Singh AK. Grid-connected and off-grid solar photovoltaic system. In: Islam F, Mamun K, Amanullah M, editors. Smart energy grid design for island countries. Green energy and technology. Cham: Springer; 2017.
6. AROS Solar Technology. Sirio power supply [online]. Aros, Cormano; 2017. Available: http://www.aros-solar.com/en/ sirio-power-supply-sps
7. Urmee T, Harries D, Holtorf H-G. Photovoltaics for rural electrification in developing countries. Cham: Springer; 2016.

8. Faranda R, Leva S, Maugeri V. MPPT techniques for PV systems: energetic and cost comparison. IEEE Power and Energy Society general meeting: Conversion and delivery of electrical energy in the 21st century, Pittsburgh, PA, 2008, pp. 1–6.
9. Brodd RJ. Batteries for sustainability. New York: Springer; 2013.
10. Entrade. Ensolar, UPS solar inverter [online]. Entrade, Padova; 2017. Available: http://www.entrade.it/it/category/ups-solar-inverter.html

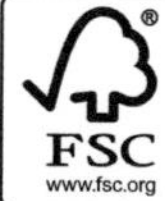